RUBELLA

Publication Number 867

AMERICAN LECTURE SERIES®

A Monograph in

The BANNERSTONE DIVISION *of*
AMERICAN LECTURES IN CLINICAL MICROBIOLOGY

Edited by

ALBERT BALOWS, Ph.D.

Chief, Bacteriology Branch
Laboratory Division
Center for Disease Control
Atlanta, Georgia

RUBELLA

FIRST ANNUAL SYMPOSIUM
OF THE EASTERN PENNSYLVANIA BRANCH
AMERICAN SOCIETY FOR MICROBIOLOGY

Edited by

HERMAN FRIEDMAN, Ph.D.

Department of Microbiology
Albert Einstein Medical Center
Philadelphia, Pennsylvania

and

JAMES E. PRIER, D.V.M., Ph.D.

Director, Division of Laboratories,
Pennsylvania Department of Health

and

Adjunct Professor of Microbiology
Temple University School of Medicine
Philadelphia, Pennsylvania

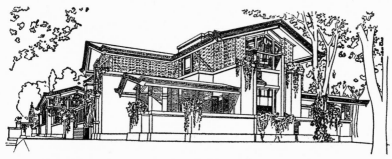

CHARLES C THOMAS · PUBLISHER
Springfield · Illinois · U.S.A.

Published and Distributed Throughout the World by
CHARLES C THOMAS • PUBLISHER
BANNERSTONE HOUSE
301-327 East Lawrence Avenue, Springfield, Illinois, U.S.A.

© *1973, by* CHARLES C THOMAS • PUBLISHER
ISBN 0-398-02650-5

Library of Congress Catalog Card Number: 72 87001

With THOMAS BOOKS *careful attention is given to all details of
manufacturing and design. It is the Publisher's desire to present books
that are satisfactory as to their physical qualities and artistic possibilities
and appropriate for their particular use.* THOMAS BOOKS *will be true
to those laws of quality that assure a good name and good will.*

Printed in the United States of America
C-1

Conference Chairman

James E. Prier, D.V.M., Ph.D.

Co-sponsored by

Flow Laboratories;
Department of Microbiology,
Temple University
School of Medicine;
Department of Microbiology,
Hahnemann School of Medicine

Contributors

Smith, Kline and French Laboratories
Bio-Screen Laboratories
Cooke Engineering Company

CONTRIBUTORS

CHARLES A. ALFORD, JR., M.D.

Medical College of Alabama
Birmingham, Alabama

LOUIS Z. COOPER, M.D.

New York University School of Medicine
New York, New York

ROBERT J. FERLAUTO, B.S.

Smith, Kline & French Laboratories
Philadelphia, Pennsylvania

KENNETH L. HERRMANN, Ph.D.

Center for Disease Control
Atlanta, Georgia

DOROTHY M. HORSTMANN, M.D.

Yale University School of Medicine
New Haven, Connecticut

ALFRED L. KALODNER, M.D.

Temple University Medical Center
Philadelphia, Pennsylvania

EDWIN H. LENNETTE, M.D., Ph.D.

Division of Laboratories
California Department of Public Health
Berkeley, California

ROBERT MacCREADY, M.D.

Windham College
Putney, Vermont

vii

HARRY M. MEYER, JR., M.D.

*National Institutes of Health
Bethesda, Maryland*

PAUL D. PARKMAN, M.D.

*National Institutes of Health
Bethesda, Maryland*

STANLEY PLOTKIN, M.D.

*The Wistar Institute of Anatomy and Biology
Philadelphia, Pennsylvania*

JAMES E. PRIER, D.V.M., Ph.D.

*Pennsylvania Department of Health
Division of Laboratories
Philadelphia, Pennsylvania*

JAY E. SATZ, Ph.D.

*Pennsylvania Department of Health
Division of Laboratories
Philadelphia, Pennsylvania*

GILBERT M. SCHIFF, M.D.

*University of Cincinnati
College of Medicine
Cincinnati, Ohio*

JOSEPH STOKES, JR., M.D.

*University of Pennsylvania
School of Medicine
Philadelphia, Pennsylvania*

CYRIL H. WECHT, M.D., LL.B.

*Medical Examiner, Allegheny County
Director, Pathology and Toxicology Laboratories
Pittsburgh, Pennsylvania*

FOREWORD

THE genesis of *American Lectures in Clinical Microbiology* stems from the concerted efforts of the Editor and the Publisher to provide a forum from which well-qualified and distinguished authors may present, either as a book or monograph, their views on any aspect of clinical microbiology. Our definition of clinical microbiology is conceived to encompass the broadest aspects of medical microbiology not only as it is applied to the clinical laboratory but equally to the research laboratory and to theoretical considerations. In the clinical microbiology laboratory we are concerned with differences in morphology, biochemical behavior and antigenic patterns as a means of microbial identification. In the research laboratory or when we employ microorganisms as a model in theoretical biology, our interest is often focused not so much on the above differences but rather on the similarities between microorganisms. However, it must be appreciated that even though there are many similarities between cells, there are important differences between major types of cells which set very definite limits on the cellular behavior. Unless this is understood it is impossible to discern common denominators.

We are also concerned with the relationships between microorganism and disease—any microorganism and any disease. Implicit in these relations is the role of the host which forms the third arm of the triangle: microorganism, disease and host. In this series we plan to explore each of these; singly where possible for factual information and in combination for an understanding of the myriad of interrelationships that exist. This necessitates the application of basic principles of biology and may, at times, require the emergence of new theoretical concepts which will create new principles or modify existing ones. Above all, our aim is to present well-documented books which will be informative, instructive and useful, creating a sense of satisfaction to both the reader and the author.

ix

Closely intertwined with the above raison d'etre is our desire to produce a series which will be read not only for the pleasure of knowledge but which will also enhance the reader's professional skill and extend his technical ability. *American Lectures in Clinical Microbiology* is dedicated to biologists—be they physicians, scientists or teachers—in the hope that this series will foster better appreciation of mutual problems and help close the gap between theoretical and applied microbiology.

This book is the outgrowth of The Annual Symposium Series of the Eastern Pennsylvania Branch of the American Society for Microbiology. The timeliness and importance of the topic—*rubella*—and the significant contributions of the participants unmistakably pointed to the need to publish the proceedings of this conference. While rubella is an old disease, our insight has deepened because of the advances in laboratory technology that permit accurate diagnosis of infection and the introduction of vaccines which now make it possible to control rubella. Dr. Prier and Dr. Friedman recognized the value of bringing together scientists and clinicians for the free exchange of information and knowledge on rubella and then to edit the presentations so that this volume rightfully takes its place in our series. A glance at the table of contents, the listing of distinguished authors and relevance of the presentations indicate why we are justified in the pride with which this volume is made available to physicians and scientists.

ALBERT BALOWS, Ph.D., *Editor*

PREFACE

A SYMPOSIUM, regardless of subject, is not an easy affair to organize and execute. It requires the labor and talents of many, and the Eastern Pennsylvania Branch of ASM has been fortunate in finding such people in their membership, and among the cooperating organizations. The Flow Laboratories were of particular help, not only in providing skilled personnel, but also in guaranteeing the financial security of the symposium. Commercial organizations, listed elsewhere, also were generous in their contribution.

If any single person could be identified as being responsible for the success of the first symposium, it certainly would be Miss Josephine Bartola, member of the local ASM Branch, and staff member of the Division of Laboratories, Pennsylvania Department of Health. Her remarkable capacity for organizing, and at the same time giving attention to a variety of complex details, has earned her the gratitude of all who were concerned with the meeting.

HERMAN FRIEDMAN
JAMES E. PRIER

CONTENTS

RUBELLA

Chapter 1

RUBELLA: VITAL PROBLEMS REMAINING

Joseph Stokes, Jr.

MORE recent pediatric immunization with live viruses may be considered as a developing mirror of nature. While small-pox vaccination may well benefit from further study of attenuation, on the other hand measles and mumps live virus vaccines have reached a fairly stable state of development that resembles nature and yet mitigates the more severe aspects of both natural diseases. Chickenpox and rubella also share the distinction of being single antigenic types that usually produce permanent immunity under natural conditions. Little is known about artificial immunization in chickenpox, while by contrast rubella live virus vaccine appears to be well on the way toward joining measles and mumps vaccines in mirroring the permanent immunizations these natural diseases have almost always produced.

In opening this symposium it would hardly seem worthwhile to review the many aspects of the clinical disease and its teratogenic consequences that suddenly sprang into prominence with Sir Norman Gregg's farsighted suggestion in 1941 concerning the probable crippling effects of rubella on the fetus during the first trimester of pregnancy. The full clinical significance of fetal infection was not realized until the aftermath of the 1964 outbreak of the disease. All of these effects, and studies on the cultivation of the virus on tissue cultures, virus attenuation, laboratory tests for detection of antibody and the variety of cells used for production of vaccine all have been detailed in the Proceedings of the International Conference on Rubella Immunization of 1969 and will be reviewed so thoroughly at the present conference that I will leave these areas to succeeding speakers. Therefore, I wish to outline certain aspects of rubella immunization that seem particularly appropriate for this conference to consider, even though

3

the data for their complete solution may not as yet be available. These aspects are as follows:

1. The theoretical possibility that the presence of rubella virus in the throats of vaccinees may be a threat to the susceptible mother during her first trimester of pregnancy.

2. The theoretical possibility that the vaccinee, when later exposed by chance to natural rubella, will respond by sufficient infection with the natural virus to pose a similar threat to the susceptible mother.

3. The theoretical possibility that the female vaccinee, when pregnancy eventuates at a considerably later date combined with exposure to natural rubella during the first trimester, may suffer sufficient infection with the natural virus to cause crippling disease in the fetus.

4. The important problem which differs in every governmental unit in this country, namely to get sufficient children vaccinated before puberty to dry up the reservoir of rubella virus in the general population and thus eliminate all actual, as well as theoretical, threats to the susceptible mother.

It should be emphasized that the first three problems are clearly considered as theoretical ones, since all of the evidence to date assembled by expert groups both from this country, as well as from abroad, would suggest that they are not actual problems.

In the first-mentioned theoretical possibility, considerable data are now available that demonstrate no evidence for transmission of the attenuated vaccine virus (at least of the HPV 77 5 duck virus) from the throat of the vaccinated child to the susceptible mother. Except perhaps for the conditions existing in a closely crowded ward for the youngest retarded children, there is no more intimate contact than that between mother and child in the home. Among 33 mothers and one nurse proven susceptible by serologic tests, we found no positive clinical or serologic evidence of cross-infection to the adult susceptibles from vaccinated children to whom the adults were intimately exposed in the home. Other workers have had similarly negative findings in small numbers of exposed susceptibles. Either the degree of attenuation or the small amount of virus excreted into the throat of the vaccinee, or perhaps both, are responsible for the absence of transmission of the attenuated virus from the vaccinee to the susceptible contact.

As opposed to the more readily transmitted viruses of chickenpox and measles that initiate epidemics every three to four years, the epidemics of rubella occur at approximately double this interval, at about six to nine years. This interval strongly suggests that the virus is not as readily transmitted as in chickenpox and measles. For example, for measles the childbearing female population is approximately 98 percent immune while for rubella approximately 17 to 20 percent of the fertile female population is susceptible, even though as children they may be considered to have lived under the same home and school environments. It would be difficult to account for these differences other than by virtue of some differences in the nature or available quantity of virus, or perhaps in factors related to both the character of the virus, as well as the quantity.

The second theoretical and equally important possibility that vaccinees may act as transmitters of the natural virus with which they may later be infected is not yet supported by significant evidence. It is true that natural virus at times can infect a vaccinee and cause an anamnestic response. Thus in the study by Grayston *et al* in Taiwan, natural virus was isolated from the throats of vaccinees. However, such virus was isolated during the first weeks after vaccination and therefore before the vaccinee would have had the opportunity to acquire a full immune response to the vaccine. Recent studies by Meyer indicate that the amount of virus secreted from the throat of previously vaccinated children who are superinfected with natural virus is so small in amount as to be of no significance. It seems clear that superinfection of previously vaccinated children constitutes no significant reservoir for spread of the natural virus. Hence, there is every indication that the objective of a national program for child immunization to eradicate the reservoir of infection for the sake of the adult woman can be realized.

The third theoretical possibility that a previously vaccinated mother, subsequently pregnant in the first trimester, might be infected with natural rubella virus during an outbreak of the disease and thereby expose her fetus to crippling infection also would appear to remain theoretical. Although natural virus would be expected to produce an anamnestic response in the mother if such exposure occurred, even to the extent of virus appearing in the throat, it would be consistent with the experience gained with measles and thus far with rubella, that in the presence of neutralizing antibody viremia does not occur and thus infection of the fetus through the placenta would not take place.

It should be clearly understood that these three theoretical considerations in no way lessen the value, importance and urgency of attacking the reservoir of rubella virus in the child population. Were any one of them by later study demonstrated to be actual, rather than theoretical, it would not vitiate a vaccination program aimed at eliminating such a reservoir. In toto, they could only limit, to a minor extent, a more complete eradication. Any such theoretical lack of complete control of the disease also appears to be of little consequence in the light of other epidemiologic evidence favoring vaccination. It was well demonstrated many years ago, by Dr. Richard Shope, that in a severe and readily transmitted respiratory disease, swine influenza, when 50 percent of a herd of swine had been vaccinated with killed swine influenza virus vaccine, the disease failed to spread through the closely crowded herd. When one-third of the herd was thus vaccinated, the disease would spread quite readily.

Rubella would appear to be less readily transmitted than influenza. In our experience with measles, when about one-half of the child population was vaccinated, the diminution in rate of the infection appeared to be considerably greater than could be accounted for by the numbers of vaccinated children alone. In other words, in both swine influenza and measles the vaccine initiated its control of these diseases well before total immunity of the population at risk.

The fourth problem mentioned, the active eradication of the childhood reservoir, depends primarily upon the determination of the general practitioners, pediatricians and public health officers to do just that—to eradicate—and secondarily, upon sufficient pressure being exerted by these groups upon the city, state and national governments for allocation of the necessary funds. This effort and allocation will vary among governmental units and among medical groups but the facts should be widely disseminated and the appropriate efforts should be expended before the next widespread outbreak occurs.

It would also be helpful to have more than one licensed vaccine on the market for the sake of competition and for assurance that the child population will be adequately covered. Sufficient problems have already arisen in vaccinating women who, at the time of vaccination, were unaware of their pregnancy.

In summation, there remains no sound evidence that the rubella vaccinee transmits attenuated virus to susceptible contacts. There also is no reason to presume that superinfection of the rubella vaccinee with natural virus permits natural infection of susceptible contacts and there is no evidence that the previously vaccinated woman, exposed during later pregnancy to natural virus, would transmit such virus to her fetus.

There is, however, mounting evidence that routine rubella vaccination of adult women poses insuperable difficulties not only for the vaccinee with a pregnancy unrecognized until after vaccination but for physicians and public health authorities alike. Thus, in view of the strong evidence favoring attenuated rubella vaccine for children, as opposed to adults, efforts should be pursued and accelerated to eliminate insofar as possible the reservoir of susceptible children in order to avoid an epidemic of rubella that may otherwise occur within the next few years. In the succeeding presentations, these matters will be fully reviewed and some answers to the fourth problem of distribution and application will be presented.

Chapter 2

THE RUBELLA HEMAGGLUTINATION-INHIBITION TEST

Louis Z. Cooper

IT is the intent of this discussion of the rubella HI antibody test to attempt to provide some perspective concerning this diagnostic procedure. This perspective is that of research clinicians whose primary concern is the elimination of the rubella problem. So, this approach is not the point of view of a person running a diagnostic laboratory or a clinician or as a public health official concerned with a vaccine program, but rather that of a team of physicians and laboratory people whose primary concern is elimination of the rubella problem. For this reason, though certainly we have to discuss buffers, pH's and red blood cells, we will not dwell on these aspects of the test.

The need for a reliable, reproducible, sensitive, inexpensive and rapid test for rubella antibody is quite evident. This is especially critical and always has been with regard to the problems that occur when a pregnant woman develops or is exposed to a rash illness. The issue has become even more critical now that rubella virus vaccines have been licensed for general use. It is quite clear that we would not have licensed rubella virus vaccine today if it had not been for the availability of the rubella HI antibody test, for it would have taken many times longer to have completed the necessary trials for evaluation of these preparations.

The report in early 1967 by Stewart and his colleagues from the Division of Biologic Standards of the development of a successful HI antibody test attributed success to (1) the use of high-titer inocula in systems which would grow rubella virus to high titer, (2) the use of serum treated for the removal of nonspecific inhibitors of hemagglutination, and (3) the selection of a sensitive red cell for the test. There was widespread acceptance of and

8

a rush by investigators by commercial interests and hospital laboratories to use this test. Those of us who had suffered with the neutralization test and its problems over the years since it was first described in 1962, would take any avenue that would eliminate the laborious task that neutralizations represented. Furthermore, the HI test was described just shortly after the successful attenuation of HPV 77 strain rubella vaccine, so there were multiple reasons for using a new, sensitive and reliable rubella antibody test. That rubella hemagglutination-inhibition was a feasible procedure and was not limited just to the circumstances described by Stewart and co-workers was quickly confirmed by other investigators using a variety of systems.

However, it was not long after the general application of this test that a period of disenchantment occurred for many of us. In our own experience, this disenchantment came in the following way: We were engaged in studies of rubella virus vaccines in which we obtained serial, sometimes daily blood specimens from vaccinees. In order to maintain objectivity, in our team Dr. Joan Giles did the clinical work, our laboratory did the laboratory testing and Dr. Saul Krugman who is responsible for our programs kept all the codes. We would complete our work with the rubella serology, go to Dr. Krugman to break the codes and then there would be a period of great disappointment, because although, in general, the results were reliable enough to tell us whether somebody developed antibody or not, we would see skips in the results. Sometimes we might break a code which would consist of serial bleedings from twelve or sixteen vaccinees and control subjects, with perhaps ten or twelve bloods from each child, and everything would be clean. Children would have no antibody, then they would seroconvert and the conversion would stay up. Other times, we would see in the midst of serial specimens from a single subject who had no detectable antibody, a specimen with an antibody titer of 1:32. It became obvious to us that we had a problem of reliability and reproductibility.

It became increasingly clear to us that other people were having this problem as well. I might give you some practical and concrete illustrations of the kinds of problems I mean. First, from our own laboratory, is the problem of how you interpret a less than 1:8 or a plus and minus 1:8 result. One of our patients, a young physician with an antibody titer that was sometimes less than 1:8, sometimes 1:8, when vaccinated did not seroconvert. I think this merely illustrates the difficulty in interpreting low level antibody titers. In all probability, this young woman has low level rubella antibody. I do not believe there is any solution to this problem, but I do not think it's a major problem. The kinds of mistakes one makes in misdiagnosis by not picking up small amounts of antibody are generally not serious. The converse is not true.

Let me illustrate a more difficult problem which we face regularly. A pregnant woman was exposed to her daughter who was exposed to a child with alleged rubella. A blood specimen was taken and was sent to a hospital laboratory where antibody titers were being done using a commercially available kit. Another blood specimen was obtained two weeks later. The first specimen was reported as no antibody at 1:10, the lowest test dilution, the second one two weeks later, at 1:80. The woman was scheduled for a therapautic abortion. The obstetrician was uneasy about this since the lady never had a rash and neither did her daughter. He referred her to us for reevaluation. In our laboratory, first of all we were unable to obtain the sera that had been run previously by the other laboratory because they had been discarded. In serum obtained by our laboratory, this lady had no detectable rubella antibody. To make a long story short, she continued to have no detectable antibody. It was suggested that she continue with her pregnancy, and she delivered a normal child without any manifestations of congenital rubella. This is an illustration of administrative and technical problems. Sera should not be discarded in circumstances such as these. This is an administrative issue. The technical problem was inadequate removal of non-specific inhibitors of hemagglutination.

Another woman was exposed to a child with a rash, blood specimens were sent two days later to a commercial laboratory and another specimen was obtained two and a half weeks later. The first titer reported was 1:160; the second two and a half weeks later, 1:640; a fourfold rise. The interpretation was "rubella." Again our unit was asked to become involved, this laboratory saved the sera and in our laboratory the titers were 1:1024 on both occasions, no rise. Furthermore, when we examined the blood of the child who allegedly was the index case, as is frequently the case, this child who was three years old had no detectable rubella antibody. Her rash illness was not rubella. This case illustrates three things: (1) again, the problem of reproducibility, a fourfold rise that wasn't a fourfold rise; (2) inadequate understanding of the natural history and immune responses of rubella; (3) a failure to use adequate epidemiological clues.

I could give other illustrations, but I think these two cases give you some idea of why we and many other people have become increasingly concerned about the use and abuse of the rubella HI antibody test, and why I say there has been a period of disenchantment with the laboratory procedure.

When one looks at these problems, they appear to have a common thread or common threads. The first group could be lumped into what I call technical difficulties and the second, poor interpretation of test results due to basic ignorance of the natural history of the immunology and the epidemiology of rubella. That second category, namely, poor interpretation due to ignorance, I think has two causes: (1) the state of the art, the fact that there are many unanswered questions concerning rubella immunology and epidemiology (I know that other participants in this symposium will address themselves to these points); (2) poor dissemination of information. The questions that are asked by people who are allegedly delivering service to physicians in terms of rubella antibody testing are appalling and frightening. It is no wonder that we have a long list of examples of the kind reported to you.

Technical difficulties can be grouped into several categories. First of all, to do reasonable rubella antibody testing and to give answers, there must be accurate and detailed histories. Otherwise, we cannot interpret the results. Many laboratories hamstring themselves by failure to insist upon adequate histories. Second is the insistence on clear labeling of specimens with clear identification in terms of name or number and proper date. We have seen terrible problems because of this. Third is the need to run serial specimens in the same test. These are biological tests and it is inconceivable that anyone could expect them to be so reproducible that you could run them individually. Fourth is the need to save sera for a prolonged period of time, at least six or eight months. It is the natural history of problems of rubella in pregnancy, for example, that women or their obstetricians are not sure when they will need another specimen. Laboratories should have the capability of saving diagnostic sera until the issue is resolved in one way or another.

Another problem is both administrative and technical, incompatibility of different techniques and different kits. Laboratories sometimes buy reagents from one company and then additional reagents from another. These usually do not match in consistency. Using leftover reagent with fresh reagent, even from the same company also is hazardous.

Finally, the problem of report forms—I am really not sure that I have seen a single adequate report form for rubella antibody testing. None seem to cover all of the circumstances. In interpretation of results, we have done as much harm as we have in inaccuracy in the test itself.

What about more precise technical problems. Of course, there have been a whole range of reports on what happens with various buffers, pH's, times and temperatures of incubation and the like; but the biggest problem has occurred with regard to pretreatment of sera for removal of nonspecific inhibitors of hemagglutination. The National Communicable Disease Center has been working for some months in an attempt to find out what are the variables that cause problems in rubella antibody testing and in an attempt to determine a standardized procedure. In the course of numerous committee meetings with people asked to participate by NCDC, much information about the variables of rubella antibody testing has been examined. Though there is not complete agreement as yet, certain features of the test are fairly well agreed upon by most persons. It is clear that although kaolin is an acceptable and useful means of removing nonspecific inhibitor and works with great accuracy in the hands of some people, in the hands of other people, including ourselves and especially the hands of the casual user, it is unreliable. Kaolin specifically removes immunoglobulin and, upon occasion, fails to remove inhibitor. Many people have moved toward the utilization of some other means of removing nonspecific inhibitor.

Manganous chloride-heparin has been reported as being effective by a number of people. In our own experience, when we attempted to use quantities such as that described initially by Mann for reovirus, manganaous chloride-heparin was ineffective. With juggling of concentrations of these reagents, one can adequately, regularly and reliably remove the beta-lipoprotein nonspecific inhibitors. Dr. Liebhaber will talk later in the session about dextran-sulfate and calcium chloride, another effective means of inhibitor removal. This important area needs further investigation.

Absorption of nonspecific serum hemagglutinins by cells raises the question of the type and concentration of cells. It is clear that a number of cells, not only the unfed chick, but pigeon and goose for example are effective for this purpose. A problem in addition to the type and specie of cell, is the stability of cell. It is fair to say that for practical purposes, chick erythrocytes have to be fresh. In our own laboratory, we can not keep chick cells more than a week. My guess is that two weeks is the limit in anybody's laboratory, depending on how careful the people are in preparing the cell.

Antigen appears to be a critical factor. There is great variability in antigens. Dr. Schmidt, Dr. Lennette and their co-workers, by using antigens with paired sera, demonstrated seroconversion or what appeared to be seroconversion but with other antigens and the same paired sera; negative results were obtained.

Despite these problems, what can be expected in the reasonable future for rubella antibody testing? It is quite clear that we can standardize the chemical, physical and temporal aspects of the test. In terms of narrowing down the biological variables so that their effects will be minimal, I think we need to know a bit more about antigens, cells and the test sera. Despite all this, we have a useful test with wide applicability.

What about interpretation or poor interpretation due to lack of knowledge? I know that others will discuss the immune response in greater detail, but I think some will be useful repetition. First of all, the question of no antibody or antibody at the lowest test dilution must be considered; by and large, we can equate this with susceptibility to infection and no past history of infection, but it must be realized that many persons who had rubella in the remote past may have no detectable antibody. It is just a question of rise, how high and when, and what kind of antibody in the primary response. After onset of rash, antibody rise is quite prompt. A matter of a day or two's delay in obtaining one's specimens may make it difficult to show significant rises. It is important to recognize that during these first few days it is easy in a primary response to demonstrate specific rubella IgM antibody. In our hands the use of 2-mercaptoethanol technic is quite effective in this time period because there are large quantities of rubella specific IgM and small quantities of IgG. After four or five days when there is more rubella IgG and less IgM the usefulness of 2-mercaptoethanol decreases quite rapidly.

What about the shape of the rubella HI antibody persistence curve? Although it is clear from our 6- to 7-year follow-up that many people maintain rubella antibodies in a fairly straight line; others demonstrate a gradual decline, occasionally to levels below the lowest serum dilution in general use (i.e. less than 1:8).

This antibody decline to undetectable levels may help explain some apparent rubella vaccine "failures." Some of the people we label as "susceptible" because we can not find antibody may have a small quantity of rubella antibody or at least some form of rubella immunity due to infection in the remote past. It is not necessary to have detectable rubella antibody to change a response when exposed to rubella from a primary response to a booster response. We have had the experience of vaccinating people with a poor vaccine, not getting any detectable antibody response but then on reimmunization having them respond with a boost rather than a primary response. I am sure others will elaborate on primary versus reinfection and primary versus booster responses.

Let us now consider the rubella HI test in diagnosis of congenital rubella. Many newborns have rubella IgM but most do not have a significant amount. Usually this antibody cannot be detected with 2-mercaptoethanol because there is so much maternal rubella specific IgG present in the newborn infant's serum. This is a point which must be stressed. Rubella IgM may be detected with other technics such as in sucrose density gradient, but 2-mercaptoethanol is of no value in demonstrating rubella IgM in cord serum.

Another important point, which Dr. Plotkin has told me for years, is that children with congenital rubella lose their antibody. In the past, I have always said "No they don't." It is quite clear now from our longitudinal study of several hundred children that as the children reach five years of age, some have lost detectable quantities of rubella antibody. This is of importance in relation to when they do or do not need vaccination and whether vaccination might be a means of detecting or making a diagnosis of congenital rubella. Preliminary experience has indicated that children with congenital rubella who have become seronegative fail to respond to rubella vaccination. This sharp contrast to the high seroconversion rate when normal seronegative children are vaccinated (approximately 98%) is most provocative from a scientific point of view and may be a useful diagnostic tool.

Where do we really stand in the matter of rubella routine serology? When you look at the things that count, namely, the state of the art, personnel, costs, money and organization, it is not a gloomy picture. If we ask, what are the important uses of rubella HI antibody testing with regard to our goal of elimination of the rubella problem, the first use is screening for immunity versus susceptibility. This is of importance in determining who should receive vaccine and with regard to whether a woman is or is not at risk when she is exposed to rubella in pregnancy. Our levels of competence to answer this question are quite good with use of data from several modifications of the HI test in current use. We can tell who does not have antibody and who does have antibody. We have difficulty in interpreting low levels and when it comes to reproducibility of tests showing high titers. A titer of 1:128 may be 1:512 in the same laboratory the same day, or even 1:1024 on another day with a different antigen or batch of red cells. If this variability is not recognized, of course, it may be disastrous from the standpoint of interpretation.

What about the state of the art with regard to the diagnosis of rash illness, exposure to rash illness or suspected congenital rubella? This is more complex and it relates to understanding the antibody response and to getting properly timed specimens. It is important for a laboratory to know when it cannot make a diagnosis because it has specimens taken at inappropriate times.

Measurement of antigenicity of vaccines is easy to do with currently available tests. The use of the HI test which, at the moment, is most difficult is in scientific investigation where a twofold or a fourfold difference in titer may be important and where antibody at a level of 1:2, 1:4 or 1:8 may be important. We have much work to do before we can talk dogmatically about reproducibility and reliability at that low level.

In terms of screening, I thought I was going to be able to tell you today of a great test that was "idiot proof," could be done on capillary or venous blood, and could be done by the hundreds in a given day. We do have such a test using specially treated filter paper discs, but we need additional quality control studies before I can label it "idiot proof." In our most recent trial, we asked a nurse who had never been in a laboratory before to run a hundred sera with this new test. She got good test results with a hundred known sera but had a good deal of spontaneous hemagglutination in the control wells. An experienced serologist could read through this for the immunes. Obviously, where there was spontaneous hemagglutination in the serum control, we could not tell if someone was truly susceptible at a 1:8 level. Nevertheless, I believe that this technique has potential for large-scale screening. We have used it already in public schools, among student nurses and in our prenatal screening program at Bellevue Hospital where 22 percent of the women who come into the prenatal clinic are now rubella susceptible. It is equally important to understand that two-thirds of rubella syndrome children are not products of first pregnancy. Therefore, even though picking patients up in their first pregnancy and vaccinating them immediately postpartum will not eliminate the rubella problem, it might decrease the problems of congenital rubella by two-thirds until "herd immunity" is well established among children.

One of our biggest difficulties is education of laboratories and consumers in terms of how to use the rubella HI antibody test and when to use the test. This meeting and the efforts of the National Communicable Disease Center are important steps toward eliminating that difficulty.

Perhaps the most important message I can try to transmit to you is my own enthusiasm that widespread availability of rubella antibody testing is feasible and important. If I can get these two points across, feasibility and importance, then in many of the sessions that go on throughout the next two days and subsequently after we leave here the few remaining technical problems *can* be and will be resolved.

Chapter 3

NEUTRALIZATION, FLUORESCENT ANTIBODY AND COMPLEMENT FIXATION TESTS FOR RUBELLA

EDWIN H. LENNETTE and NATHALIE J. SCHMIDT

THE hemagglutination-inhibition (HI) test for rubella is now the most widely used serologic procedure for the diagnosis of rubella infections and for determination of immune status. It is a highly sensitive method for the detection of rubella antibody and is the most practical serologic test available from the standpoint of economy and the rapidity with which results can be obtained. However, other antibody assay methods such as the neutralization test, immunofluorescent antibody staining, and particularly the complement fixation (CF) test may also have application under certain circumstances.

NEUTRALIZATION TESTS

For the first two or three years after the initial isolation of rubella virus, the neutralization test was the only method available for antibody assays. One of the difficulties encountered in the development of neutralizing antibody assays for rubella is the fact that neutralization of this virus is difficult to demonstrate, and low test doses of virus must be employed, making reproducibility of results difficult to achieve. The first assays for neutralizing antibody to rubella virus were based on the interference technique (1-3), a method influenced by the variables of both the rubella and challenge virus systems. Some of the variables found to influence the test system most profoundly were the

From the Viral and Rickettsial Disease Laboratory, California State Department of Public Health, Berkeley, California 94704.

The work on which this paper is based was supported in part by Grant AI-01475 from the National Institute of Allergy and Infectious Diseases, National Institutes of Health, United States Public Health Service, Department of Health, Education and Welfare.

18

test dose of rubella virus employed, the use of heated or un-heated test serum, the preliminary incubation of serum-virus mixtures prior to inoculation into cell cultures, and the length of time which cultures were incubated before addition of the challenge virus. In addition to the number of variables in the test system, other drawbacks to the use of interference neutralization tests are the extra manipulations involved in adding the challenge virus and the length of time required before results are obtainable, usually ten to fourteen days.

Despite the problems encountered in reproducing the results of antibody quantitation, wide experience obtained with the interference neutralization test during the recent rubella outbreak showed it to be a reliable technique for determining the immunity status of individuals (presence or absence of antibody) and for demonstrating diagnostically significant increases in antibody levels.

Neutralizing antibody assays based upon inhibition of the direct cytopathic effect of laboratory-adapted strains of rubella virus in certain rabbit cell lines (4-7) have simplified the test procedure and have, in some instances, shortened the length of time required for results to be obtained. Recently a micro-method has been described for assay of rubella neutralizing antibodies (8).

The precision of rubella neutralizing antibody assays has been increased by the development of plaque-reduction tests. In these test systems, plaques may be demonstrated by the hemadsorption-negative procedure using Newcastle disease virus for challenge (9), by the direct cytopathic effect of the virus under a solid over-lay (10, 11) or by the hemadsorption of pigeon erythrocytes onto foci (plaques) of rubella-infected cells (12). Although rubella neutralizing antibody titers demonstrated by plaque reduction have not been markedly higher than those obtained in interference neutralization tests, reproducibility is generally greater, due to less influence of variations in the test dose of virus, and results are usually obtained earlier than in tests based on interference or development of cytopathic effects.

A number of investigators have shown that, as is true of a number of other viruses, neutralization of rubella virus is enhanced by an "accessory factor" present in fresh, unheated serum (2, 3,

5, 9), and in some neutralization tests for rubella antibody, the test serum is not inactivated (4, 13). In general, however, since the amount of accessory factor present may vary from serum to serum, and may also be decreased by storage at 4°C, it is considered more desirable to inactivate the test serum and then to restore the enhancing factor through the addition of a standard amount of fresh, normal serum. Fresh rabbit, guinea pig and horse sera have all been shown capable of enhancing neutralization of rubella virus (2, 3, 14), but rabbit serum is reportedly inconsistent in this respect (13, 14), and indeed certain lots of normal rabbit and guinea pig serum have been found to possess inhibitory activity for rubella virus.

Findings recently reported by Almeida (15) shed some light on the possible mechanism underlying enhancement of rubella virus neutralization by fresh serum. She has shown, by electron microscopic examination of rubella virus aggregated by specific antisera, that the outer coat of the virus is lysed in aggregates produced by unheated sera, while in aggregates produced by heated sera the morphology of the virus is intact. Thus, it appears that with fresh serum, antibody and complement exert a virolytic effect which enhances the neutralizing activity of the antiserum.

Although the neutralization test is a highly sensitive method for detecting rubella antibody induced by current or past infections, its diagnostic usefulness is limited by the fact that neutralizing antibody appears very early in the course of infection and may be at maximum levels by the time the acute-phase serum specimen is collected, making it impossible to demonstrate a diagnostically significant increase in antibody titer over the course of the illness. Table 3-I shows the results of a comparison conducted in our laboratory on the relative diagnostic value of neutralization, complement fixation, fluorescent antibody and HI tests for rubella. The paired sera were from 99 cases of suspected rubella on whom acute-phase sera were collected during the first seven days after onset and convalescent-phase sera were collected fourteen or more days after onset of infection. Rubella neutralizing antibody was demonstrable in the sera of 84 of these individuals, but significant increases in antibody were shown for only 33,

TABLE 3-I

RESULTS OF NEUTRALIZATION (Neut.), COMPLEMENT FIXATION (CF), FLUORESCENT ANTIBODY (FA) AND HEMAGGLUTINATION-INHIBITION (HI) TESTS IN 99 CASES* OF SUSPECTED RUBELLA

Type of Test	Fourfold or Greater Rise in Titer	No Rise in Titer, Antibody Present	No Antibody† Demonstrable
Neut.	33	51	15
CF	48	26	25
FA	51	30	18
HI	51	30	18

* Cases with satisfactory paired sera tested; acute-phase serum collected within 7 days, convalescent-phase serum 14 or more days after onset.

† <1:4 for neut., CF and FA tests; <1:8 for HI tests. (Reproduced with permission from *J. Immunol.*, 99:785-793, 1967.)

as compared to 48 by CF, 51 by indirect fluorescent antibody (FA) and 51 by HI tests.

HI antibody also appears early in the course of infection, but it has been our experience that diagnostically significant increases in titer are more often demonstrable by this procedure than by neutralization tests. One possible explanation for this is that kaolin treatment used to remove nonspecific inhibitors from sera prior to their examination in HI tests also removes IgM from serum, and this might reduce levels of early rubella antibody, which is IgM in nature, so that an increase in titer is demonstrable between the acute-phase serum and the convalescent-phase serum containing relatively less IgM and more IgG antibody. Similarly the greater diagnostic value of the indirect FA test over the neutralization test might be due to the fact that the fluorescein-labeled anti-human globulin conjugate used for FA tests is directed largely against IgG immunoglobulins and is relatively insensitive for the detection of the early IgM antibodies.

Although neutralizing antibody assays are no longer required for routine serologic diagnosis of rubella virus infections, or for determination of immunity to rubella, they are sometimes necessary for resolution of equivocal results obtained in HI tests. In certain instances sera which fail to show antibody in HI tests do show neutralizing antibody activity. The proportion of HI-negative sera showing neutralizing antibodies for rubella has ranged from 2 to 24 percent in various studies (7, 8, 16-18). Whether this is due to removal of antibody by procedures used to remove nonspecific inhibitors from sera prior to HI testing, or to a greater sensitivity of neutralizing antibody assays is not clear. At any rate, with increased awareness of the need for standardization of HI antibody test procedures, neutralization tests will be required as a basis for comparison.

FLUORESCENT ANTIBODY TESTS

Indirect immunofluorescent staining techniques for assay of rubella antibodies were first described in 1964. Brown and associates (19) employed chronically infected cell cultures of the LLC-MK₂ rhesus monkey kidney line as a source of antigen for staining, while Schaeffer and co-workers (20) utilized infected primary cultures of African green monkey kidney cells. Serial dilutions of the test serum are applied to fixed virus-infected cells, and if antibody is present its union with virus in the cells is detected through the use of fluorescein-labeled anti-human immune globulins.

Although the indirect fluorescent antibody (FA) technique offered a much simpler and more rapid method than the neutralization test for assay of rubella antibody, attempts to use the procedure on a large-scale diagnostic basis met with varying degrees of success. One of the major problems in performing FA assays for rubella is that of obtaining infected cells containing large amounts of antigen. The sensitivity of the technic is also dependent upon the use of high-titered and specific anti-human globulin conjugates.

In our laboratory a modified indirect immunofluorescent staining technique has been developed for assay of rubella antibodies (21). This procedure proved to be as sensitive as neutralization tests for detection of antibody and more reliable than neutralization tests for demonstrating diagnostically significant increases in antibody titer (17, 21, 22). Smears of rubella-infected cells are employed for staining rather than infected coverslip cultures. Initially the BS-C-1 line of grivet monkey kidney cells was employed, and more recently the BHK-21 line of baby hamster kidney cells has been found to be very satisfactory. With either cell line it is important to infect the cells with a large dose of virus to obtain maximum numbers of infected cells for staining. Nonspecific staining and overstaining has been reduced by preparing test serum dilutions and conjugate dilutions in 20% suspension of beef brain, and also by centrifuging sera or passing them through a Millipore filter prior to testing.

Another difference between our FA procedure and those described by other investigators is that antibody endpoints are expressed in terms of the highest initial dilution of serum giving clear-cut staining rather than the highest dilution giving 3-plus or 4-plus staining. Endpoints based upon this type of reading have been found to be reproducible, and readings are less subjective than those based upon gradations of fluorescence. Rubella antigen is located in the cytoplasm of infected cells, and it has a fine, granular appearance; in many cells it fills the cytoplasm. Glaring (4+) fluorescence is rarely seen. Convalescent-phase sera from individuals with a rubella infection generally give 2-plus to 3-plus staining in the lower serum dilutions, diminishing to 1-plus reactions at the 1:64 to 1:128 dilutions.

Antibody titers obtained by our FA procedure are usually somewhat higher than those observed in neutralization tests, but other investigators have reported FA titers to be similar to or lower than neutralizing antibody titers (18, 23-25). Titer levels depend not only upon the procedure employed, but also upon the endpoints selected for reading test results.

We have found the FA test to be comparable to the HI test, slightly more sensitive than the CF test, and markedly more sensitive than the neutralization test for demonstration of diagnostically significant antibody titer rises. In one comparative study (17), 90 percent of infections diagnosed by a significant increase in one or more types of antibody were positive by either FA and HI tests, while 83 percent were positive by CF and 60 percent by neutralization tests. Others (18, 23-25) have reported very similar findings for the diagnostic value of the HI, CF and neutralization tests, but found the FA test to give positive results for only 70 to 80 percent of their laboratory-confirmed cases of rubella virus infection.

Some studies have reported the FA test to be less reliable than neutralization or HI tests for detecting antibody from past infections (23-25), but in our experience the FA test is as satisfactory as the HI and neutralization tests for this purpose. The length of time antibodies demonstrated by the indirect FA test persist after infection is still uncertain. There have been reports that sera from individuals who had rubella ten or more years previously showed a fainter staining reaction than did sera from recent infections (23, 24). On the other hand, results of studies conducted by the New York State Health Department (18) suggest that immunofluorescence antibodies may persist for as long as neutralizing and HI antibodies; serial specimens collected from the same individuals at intervals over periods up to thirteen years showed no decrease in either HI or FA titers for rubella.

It has been reported (26) that individuals receiving attenuated rubella virus vaccines show a negative or very weak fluorescent antibody response, and it has been suggested that the FA test might be used in conjunction with HI tests to distinguish between antibody produced by natural infections and by vaccination.

Although the indirect FA technique has been largely supplanted by the HI test for assay of rubella antibodies, it is still useful in instances where HI tests give equivocal results; it is a simpler and more rapid method for this purpose than is the neutralization test. Laboratories offering consultative and reference services in rubella HI serology should also have expertise in the FA test so that it can be used for confirmation of results.

Of importance in the serologic diagnosis of rubella infections are the recent reports (27, 28) that IgM rubella antibody can be detected by the indirect FA technic through the use of a conjugate specific for human IgM. This serves as the basis for more rapid diagnosis of congenital infections and also for diagnosis of recent infections in which significant antibody titer rises cannot be demonstrated.

COMPLEMENT FIXATION TESTS

Complement-fixing (CF) antigens for rubella were first developed in 1964 (29-31). In order to demonstrate specific CF activity in rubella-infected cell cultures it was necessary to employ highly concentrated preparations of infected cells (29, 30) or culture fluids (31), and therefore the first CF antigens available for serologic diagnosis were costly and cumbersome to prepare. The routine application of the CF test for diagnosis of rubella infections was extended greatly by the finding that high concentrations of CF antigen are produced in the BHK-21 line of baby hamster kidney cells (32, 33) and that high-titered antigens can be produced either from the infected fluid phase of cultures or, more conveniently, by extraction of the cellular phase with alkaline buffers (33). The use of high-titered antigens derived from BHK-21 cells gives higher antibody titers in CF tests and thus results in tests of greater sensitivity.

Even though CF antigens for rubella have been, and still are, relatively costly to prepare, the CF test has contributed much to the serodiagnosis of rubella infections. Early studies showed that the CF test for rubella was highly specific, and that antibody titer rises to rubella virus did not occur in other viral infections (30, 32). The specificity of the test is further evidenced by the fact that, in testing hundreds of sera, we have encountered only a single serum which showed rubella CF activity (a low titer, 1:4) in the absence of corresponding neutralizing or HI activity.

Complement-fixing (CF) antibodies develop more slowly in the course of rubella infections than do neutralizing or HI antibodies and may not be demonstrable until two weeks after onset. This relatively slow development of CF antibody is advantageous from the standpoint of serologic diagnosis, since in some cases in which the acute-phase serum specimen is collected rather late in the course of infection, neutralizing or HI antibody levels may already be elevated and fail to show a significant increase in the convalescent-phase specimen. In these instances a significant increase can generally be demonstrated in slower-appearing CF antibody.

The combination of the HI test and the CF test has been found to be the most reliable for serologic diagnosis of rubella infections (17, 25). Table 3-II summarizes the positive serologic diagnoses of rubella infection made in our laboratory since the HI

TABLE 3-II

COMPARATIVE DIAGNOSTIC VALUE OF HI AND CF TESTS
FOR RUBELLA

No. of Patients Positive* for Rubella by Either HI or CF	No. Positive by Both Tests	No. Positive by HI only	No. Positive by CF only
229	195 (85%)	16 (7%)	18 (8%)

Tests conducted in 1967, 1968 and 1969.
* Positive = fourfold or greater rise in antibody titer between acute- and convalescent-phase serum specimens.

test was adopted on a routine basis early in 1967. It is seen that 85 percent of the patients showed significant antibody titer rises by both HI and CF tests, while 7 percent were positive only in HI tests and 8 percent were positive only by the CF test. Table 3-III summarizes the time of collection and median antibody titers of sera from those patients showing a positive reaction in only a single test. With patients positive only by HI, acute-phase sera were collected within one to three days after onset of infection, and they showed no antibody by either HI or CF tests. Convalescent-phase sera on these patients were collected early in the course of infection and, while HI antibody had reached significant levels, CF antibody had reached titers of only 1:4. In the case of infections diagnosed only by CF tests, acute-phase sera were collected relatively late and HI antibody titers were already elevated, but CF antibody was not yet demonstrable. The convalescent-phase sera for these patients did not show significant increases in HI titer, but CF titers increased fourfold or more.

TABLE 3-III

TIME OF COLLECTION AND MEDIAN ANTIBODY TITERS OF SERA
FROM RUBELLA PATIENTS SHOWING POSITIVE REACTIONS IN
ONLY A SINGLE TEST

Patient Group	Number of Patients	Acute-phase Sera Days After Onset	Median Titer HI	CF	Convalescent-phase Sera Days After Onset	Median Titer HI	CF
Positive by HI only	16	1-3	<8	<4	14-60	256	16
Positive by CF only	18	5-12	128	<4	11-19	128	4

Wherever possible the CF test should be used in addition to the HI test for laboratory diagnosis of rubella infections, since an additional 5 to 10 percent of infections which are not diagnosed by the HI test can be diagnosed by the CF test.

CF antibody declines over the years to undetectable levels, and thus the CF test is not as useful as are neutralization, FA or HI tests for determination of immunity status (17, 23-25).

It has been noted that immunization with attenuated rubella virus vaccines does not generally elicit detectable levels of CF antibody (34).

NATURE OF RUBELLA CF ANTIGENS

In addition to developing the rubella CF test as a diagnostic tool, our laboratory has also been interested in studying the basic nature of rubella CF antigens and determining the relationship of the CF antigens to the infectious viral particle and the hemagglutinin.

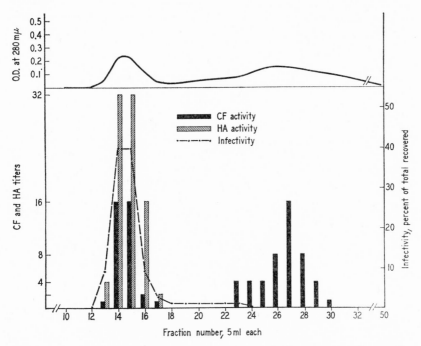

Figure 3-1. Elution of rubella antigens from Sephadex G 200 column. Reprinted with permission from *J. Immunol.*, 100:851-857, 1968.

We found that virtually all of the CF antigen in infected RK-13 (rabbit kidney) cells was soluble in nature and was not sedimented under conditions of centrifugation which sedimented the infectious viral particle (31). Using higher-titered antigens prepared in BHK-21 cells it was possible by Sephadex gel filtration to demonstrate two distinct CF antigens for rubella, one (the large particle antigen) associated with the infectious viral particle and the hemagglutinin, and a smaller, "soluble" antigen having no infectivity or HA activity (35, 36). Figure 3-1 shows the elution pattern of the antigens from Sephadex G-200. The infectivity, HA activity and part of the CF activity (large-particle or viral antigen) eluted together, just after displacement of the

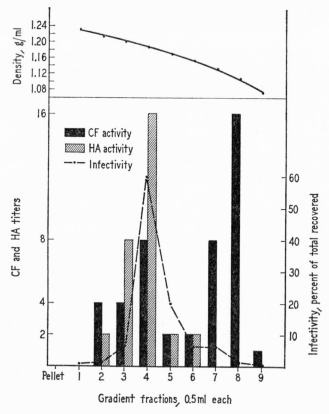

Figure 3-2. Distribution of rubella antigens in a sucrose density gradient. Reprinted with permission from *J. Immunol.*, 100:851-857, 1968.

void volume of the column, while the soluble CF antigen eluted in later fractions.

Figure 3-2 shows the results of a representative experiment in which a rubella virus preparation was centrifuged in a sucrose density gradient. The infectious virus, HA activity and large-particle CF antigen equilibrated together at densities of 1.19 to 1.21 gm/ml. The soluble (small-particle) antigen, in contrast to the soluble CF antigen of myxoviruses, was less dense than the infectious virus, and it equilibrated at densities of 1.08 to 1.10 gm/ml. Somewhat higher apparent buoyant densities were obtained for both antigens in cesium chloride density gradients.

To study the immunological properties of the viral and soluble antigens of rubella, the antigens were separated by Sephadex gel filtration and then employed for immunization of rabbits. Antibodies produced in response to viral and soluble antigens were serologically indistinguishable in CF tests, and both viral and soluble antigens elicited the formation of neutralizing and HI antibodies. This suggests that the soluble CF antigen of rubella has a protein composition identical or very similar to that of the virion, and that it is a subunit of the viral coat rather than an internal component. The immunological relationship between rubella viral and soluble antigens has also been confirmed by immunodiffusion tests (37).

REFERENCES

1. Parkman, P. D., Buescher, E. L., and Artenstein, M. S.: Recovery of rubella virus from army recruits. *Proc. Soc. Exp. Biol. Med.,* 111: 225-230, 1962.
2. Neva, F. A., and Weller, T. H.: Rubella interferon and factors influencing the indirect neutralization test for rubella antibody. *J. Immunol.,* 93:466-473, 1964.
3. Parkman, P. D., Mundon, F. K., McCown, J. M., and Buescher, E. L.: Studies of rubella. II. Neutralization of the virus. *J. Immunol.,* 93:608-617, 1964.
4. Dudgeon, J. A., Butler, N. R., and Plotkin, S. A.: Further serological studies on the rubella syndrome. *Br. Med. J.,* 2:155-160, 1964.
5. Leerhøy, J.: Neutralization of rubella virus in a rabbit cornea cell line (SIRC). *Acta Pathol. Microbiol. Scand.,* 67:158-159, 1966.
6. Hull, R. N., and Butorac, G.: The utility of rabbit kidney cell strain, LLC-RK$_1$ to rubella virus studies. *Am. J. Epidemiol.,* 83:509-517, 1966.

7. Fuccillo, D. A., Sever, J. L., Gitnick, G. L., Traub, R. G., and Huebner, R. J.: Rubella neutralizing antibody determinations with the rabbit kidney cell strain LLC-RK$_1$. *Proc. Soc. Exp. Biol. Med.,* 129:650-652, 1968.

8. Furesz, J., Moreau, P., and Yarosh, W.: A micro tissue culture test for the titration and neutralization of rubella virus. *Can. J. Microbiol.,* 15:67-71, 1969.

9. Rawls, W. E., Desmyter, J., and Melnick, J. L.: Rubella virus neutralization by plaque reduction. *Proc. Soc. Exp. Biol. Med.,* 124:167-172, 1966.

10. Vaheri, A., Sedwick, D. W., and Plotkin, S. A.: Growth of rubella virus in BHK-21 cells. I. Production, assay, and adaptation of virus. *Proc. Soc. Exp. Biol. Med.,* 125:1086-1092, 1967.

11. Rhim, J. S., Schell, K., and Huebner, R. J.: Plaque assays of rubella virus in cultures of rabbit cornea (SIRC) cells. *Proc. Soc. Exp. Biol. Med.,* 125:1271-1274, 1967.

12. Schmidt, N. J., Lennette, E. H., and Dennis, J.: A plaque assay for rubella virus based upon hemadsorption. *Proc. Soc. Exp. Biol. Med.,* 132:128-133, 1969.

13. Plotkin, S. A.: Virologic assistance in the management of German measles in pregnancy. *J.A.M.A.,* 190:105-108, 1964.

14. Leerhøy, J.: Rubella virus neutralization in heated sera. *Acta Pathol. Microbiol. Scand.,* 73:275-282, 1968.

15. Almeida, J. D.: Heated and unheated antiserum on rubella virus. *Am. J. Dis. Child.,* 118:101-106, 1969.

16. Field, A. M., Vandervelde, E. M., Thompson, K. M., and Hutchinson, D. N.: A comparison of the haemagglutination-inhibition test and the neutralization test for the detection of rubella antibody. *Lancet,* 2:182-184, 1967.

17. Lennette, E. H., Schmidt, N. J., and Magoffin, R. L.: The hemagglutination inhibition test for rubella: a comparison of its sensitivity to that of neutralization, complement fixation and fluorescent antibody tests for diagnosis of infection and determination of immunity status. *J. Immunol.,* 99:785-793, 1967.

18. Diebel, R., Cohen, S. M., and Ducharme, C. P.: Serology of rubella. Virus neutralization, immunofluorescence in BHK21 cells and hemagglutination inhibition. *N.Y. State J. Med.,* 68:1355-1362, 1968.

19. Brown, G. C., Maassab, H. F., Veronelli, J. A., and Francis, T., Jr.: Rubella antibodies in human serum: detection by the indirect fluorescent-antibody technique. *Science,* 145:943-945, 1964.

20. Schaeffer, M., Orsi, E. V., and Widelock, D.: Applications of immunofluorescence in public health virology. *Bacteriol. Rev.,* 28:402-408, 1964.

21. Lennette, E. H., Woodie, J. D., and Schmidt, N. J.: A modified in-

direct immunofluorescent staining technique for the demonstration of rubella antibodies in human sera. *J. Lab. Clin. Med.*, 69:689-695, 1967.

22. Lennette, E. H., Schmidt, N. J., and Magoffin, R. L.: Serology of rubella. Comparison of fluorescent antibody, complement fixation and neutralization tests for diagnosis of current infections and determination of sero-immunity. *Calif. Med.*, 107:223-231, 1967.

23. Sever, J. L., Huebner, R. J., Fabiyi, A., Monif, G. R., Castellano, G., Cusumano, C. L., Traub, R. G., Ley, A. C., Gilkeson, M. R., and Roberts, J. M.: Antibody responses in acute and chronic rubella. *Proc. Soc. Exp. Biol. Med.*, 122:513-516, 1966.

24. Sever, J. L., Fuccillo, D. A., Gitnick, G. L., Huebner, R. J., Gilkeson, M. R., Ley, A. C., Tzan, N., and Traub, R. G.: Rubella antibody determinations. *Pediatrics*, 40:789-797, 1967.

25. Herrmann, K. L., Halonen, P. E., Stewart, J. A., Casey, H. L., Ryan, J. M., Hall, A. D., and Caswell, K. E.: Evaluation of serological techniques for titration of rubella antibody. *Am. J. Public Health*, 59:296-304, 1969.

26. Monto, A. S., Cavallaro, J. J., and Brown, G. C.: Attenuated rubella vaccination in families: observations on the lack of fluorescent antibody response and on the use of blood collected on filter paper discs in the hemagglutination-inhibition test. *J. Lab. Clin. Med.*, 74:98-102, 1969.

27. Baublis, J. V., and Brown, G. C.: Specific response of the immunoglobulins to rubella infection. *Proc. Soc. Exp. Biol. Med.*, 128:206-210, 1968.

28. Cohen, S. M., Ducharme, C. P., Carpenter, C. A., and Deibel, R.: Rubella antibody in IgG and IgM immunoglobulins detected by immunofluorescence. *J. Lab. Clin. Med.*, 72:760-766, 1968.

29. Sever, J. L., Huebner, R. J., Castellano, G. A., Sarma, P. S., Fabiyi, A., Schiff, G. M., and Cusumano, C. L.: Rubella complement fixation test. *Science*, 148:385-387, 1965.

30. Stern, H.: Rubella virus complement-fixation test. *Nature*, 208:200-201, 1965.

31. Schmidt, N. J., and Lennette, E. H.: The complement-fixing antigen of rubella virus. *Proc. Soc. Exp. Biol. Med.*, 121:243-250, 1966.

32. Schell, K., Wong, K. T., Turner, H. C., and Huebner, R. J.: Production of rubella complement fixing antigen in BHK-21 cells. *Proc. Soc. Exp. Biol. Med.*, 123:832-836, 1966.

33. Schmidt, N. J., and Lennette, E. H.: Rubella complement-fixing antigens derived from the fluid and cellular phases of infected BHK-21 cells; extraction of cell-associated antigen with alkaline buffers. *J. Immunol.*, 97:815-821, 1966.

34. Meyer, H. M., Jr., Parkman, P. D., Hobbins, T. E., and Ennis, F. A.:

Clinical studies with experimental live rubella virus vaccine (strain HPV-77). *Am. J. Dis. Child.*, 115:648-654, 1968.

35. Schmidt, N. J., Lennette, E. H., and Gee, P. S.: Demonstration of rubella complement-fixing antigens of two distinct particle sizes by gel filtration on Sephadex G-200. *Proc. Soc. Exp. Biol. Med.*, 123: 758-762, 1966.

36. Schmidt, N. J., Lennette, E. H., Gee, P. S., and Dennis, J.: Physical and immunologic properties of rubella antigens. *J. Immunol.*, 100: 851-857, 1968.

37. Schmidt, N. J., and Styk, B.: Immunodiffusion reactions with rubella antigens. *J. Immunol.*, 101:210-216, 1968.

Chapter 4

VIRUS ISOLATION PROCEDURES

PAUL D. PARKMAN, HOPE E. HOPPS and HARRY M. MEYER, JR.

INTRODUCTION

R UBELLA virus was first isolated in 1962 by two groups of investigators working independently and using different techniques. Drs. Weller and Neva at the Harvard School of Medicine noted a subtle cytopathic effect (CPE) in primary human amnion cell cultures (1). Drs. Parkman, Buescher and Artenstein at the Walter Reed Army Institute of Research employed an interference system based on the resistance of rubella virus infected primary African green monkey kidney cells (AGMK) to challenge with enteroviruses (2). Since these original observations, other sensitive systems have been described for virus recovery of both virulent and attenuated rubella viruses. A review of these methods and their use in the study of persons experiencing rubella virus infections is presented in this report. Specimens were obtained for clinical studies from military recruits at Fort Dix, New Jersey in 1961 and 1962, from children and adults with clinical rubella in the Washington, D.C. area in 1964 and from children residing at the Arkansas Children's Colony, Conway, Arkansas in 1966-1969.

CELL CULTURES

Primary cultures of AGMK and continuous cell cultures of BS-C-1 (3), Vero (4), LLC-MK2 (5), MA-104, RK$_{13}$ (6) and BHK-21 (7) cells were obtained from the Tissue Culture Section, Division of Biologics Standards. Primary chick and duck embryo cell cultures were prepared in our laboratory. The GMK cultures were maintained at 35°C in Eagle's basal medium (BME)

From the Laboratory of Viral Immunology, Division of Biologics Standards, National Institutes of Health, Department of Health, Education and Welfare, Bethesda, Maryland 20014.

or Eagle's minimum essential medium (MEM) containing 2% chicken serum which had been heated at 56°C for 30 minutes. The RK$_{13}$ cells were incubated at 33°C and received M-199 medium containing 2% fetal bovine serum which had been similarly heat inactivated. Other cell culture types were maintained at 35°C using MEM with heat inactivated fetal bovine serum. For hemagglutinin production with freshly isolated viruses, culture medium without serum or with 2% kaolin treated fetal bovine serum was used. All culture media contained penicillin, 100 units/ml and streptomycin sulfate 100μg/ml. Culture vessels were incubated in stationary racks or trays.

Specimens for virus isolation attempts were routinely inoculated into GMK cultures. Pharyngeal swab specimens were collected with sterile cotton swabs, which were then immersed in 6 ml of BME containing 1% bovine plasma albumin, penicillin 1000 units/ml, streptomycin sulfate, 1000μg/ml and amphotericin B, 10μg/ml. In older subjects, throat washing specimens were collected by having the subject gargle with Hanks balanced salt solution (HBSS) containing 1% bovine plasma albumin. Here the penicillin, streptomycin and amphotericin B were added before inoculation of cell cultures. Blood was collected by venipuncture and heparinized (0.2 mg heparin without preservative/ml of whole blood).

Tissue specimens were weighed, ground in Ten Broeck grinders and prepared as 10% suspensions in HBSS containing 1% bovine plasma albumin and antibiotics. The swab specimens, throat washings, heparinized bloods and tissue suspensions were inoculated in 0.5 ml volumes into each of three to five AGMK tube cultures from which the medium had been removed. After an adsorption period of 1 to 2 hours, the specimen was removed, and 1 ml of maintenance medium added. The cultures were incubated at 35°C. Subpassage of pooled supernatant fluids from all of the inoculated cultures, containing cells scraped free from the glass of 2 to 4 of the tubes, were made after 10 days of incubation. Two-tenths milliliters of these pooled cells and supernatants were inoculated into each of three cultures. Both the originally inoculated and subpassage cultures were tested for the presence of interfering agents by adding approximately 1,000 tissue culture infectious doses ($TCID_{50}$) of echovirus type 11 contained in 1 ml of fresh maintenance medium. Representative interfering isolates were identified as rubella virus with specific immune serum either by neutralization or by hemagglutination inhibition of antigens prepared in BHK-21 cell cultures.

VIRUS TITRATIONS

Viruses were titrated in either AGMK or RK_{13} cell cultures. Tenfold serial dilutions of the sample were prepared in HBSS with 1% bovine plasma albumin; each dilution was inoculated in 0.1 ml volumes into five tube cultures. The cultures received fresh maintenance medium on the fifth to seventh day after infection. On the tenth day, virus infectivity was measured in AGMK cultures by interference with echovirus type 11. The RK_{13} cultures were examined for CPE after 14 days, and final readings were usually made on day 21. Fifty percent endpoints were calculated by the Karber method (8).

CULTURES USED FOR PROPAGATION OF RUBELLA VIRUS

Several of the cell lines which have been used for the propagation of rubella virus are listed in Table 4-I. It is apparent that rubella virus multiplied in many cell types; primary and continuous cultures of human, simian, and rabbit origin were found to be useful for detection of rubella virus either by CPE or interference.

The initial cytopathic system was based on the ability of the virus to produce cytopathic effects in primary human amnion cell cultures incubated for prolonged periods. Inoculated cultures showed changes characterized by the gradual appearance of CPE beginning 17 to 34 days after incubation which gradually spread to involve 50 percent or more of the cell sheet. With adaptation, viruses produced 90% cell destruction after three to five weeks. Subsequently, it was shown that such infected cultures were resistant to challenge with Sindbis virus; since this interference developed early. It was employed as an ancillary method for virus detection in this system (1). As indicated in the last column of Table 4-I, virus grown in primary amnion cells could be readily subpassaged to AGMK cultures. Primary human em-

TABLE 4-I

CELL CULTURES COMMONLY USED FOR THE GROWTH OF
RUBELLA VIRUS

Species	Cell Culture	Method of Virus Detection		
		CPE	Interference	Subpassage
Human	Primary amnion	+	+	+
	Embryo kidney	0	±*	+
	Adult thyroid	+	NT	+
	Embryonic cell strains	0	±	+
Monkey	Primary green kidney	0	+	+
	Primary patas kidney	0	+	+
	Continuous green kidney			
	BS-C-1	0	+	+
	Vero	±	0	+
	AH-1	+	NT	+
	Continuous rhesus kidney			
	MA-104	0	+	+
	LLC-MK2	±	+	+
Rabbit	Primary kidney	±	+	+
	Continuous			
	GLRK₁₃	+	NT	+
	LLC-RK1	+	NT	+
	SIRC	+	NT	+
Hamster	Continuous			
	BHK-21	±	NT	+
Avian	Primary chick embryo	0	+	+
	Primary duck embryo	0	NT	+
Canine	Primary kidney	0	NT	+

* Phenomenon inconsistent between cell culture lots.

bryo kidney supported the growth of virus but failed to show
CPE and the interference phenomenon did not consistently develop. Primary cultures of adult thyroid gland have been reported to exhibit rubella CPE (6). Growth of rubella in human
diploid cells has been shown by several workers (9, 10). Plotkin detected virus in these cells using polio virus and herpes
virus challenge but found that it was not possible to perform accurate titrations by interference.

Cells of monkey and rabbit origin have been most extensively
used for recovery and assay of rubella virus infectivity. The interference system originally reported was based on the observation that AGMK cultures inoculated with specimens collected
from patients with rubella, although remaining morphologically

normal, became totally resistant to the CPE of other viruses. The interference phenomenon became apparent in cultures inoculated with throat washings of rubella patients within 7 to 10 days. Echovirus type 11 was originally used; however, it was soon apparent that viruses in the enterovirus, arbovirus, myxovirus and papovavirus groups were also sensitive for detection of rubella virus-induced interference (9).

Using interference techniques, continuous BS-C-1 green monkey kidney, MA-104 and LLC-NK2 rhesus kidney cells have also been successfully employed (9, 11, 12). Rubella cytopathic changes in such cell lines as Vero (4, 13), AH-1 (14) and LLC-MK2 (11) have been reported. Of the simian cultures tested, only Vero cells lacked the ability to show interference. Tests in our laboratory failed to show any evidence that infected Vero cells resisted challenge with echovirus type 11, vesicular stomatitis virus, Sindbis, vaccinia and herpes virus hominis. In our hands, these cells did not produce detectable levels of interferon after infection with rubella virus. These results confirm observations of Desmyter *et al* (15).

Rabbit cells have provided an especially useful resource. Infected primary cultures show minimal cytopathic changes (16) and early, complete interference with vesicular stomatitis and Eastern equine encephalitis viruses (2). Certain continuous rabbit cell lines have shown the most prominent cytopathic changes; RK_{13} cells (6) have been widely used as well as Sirc (17) and LLC-RK1 cultures (18).

The remaining cultures listed in Table 4-I have not been used for primary isolation of virus but are included because of their special areas of usefulness. Continuous BHK-21 cells have been particularly valuable in providing high virus yields (19). Primary duck embryo (20) and canine cell cultures (21), as well as primary rabbit kidney cells (22) and WI-38 cells (23) have been employed as substrates for rubella vaccine production. Fluorescence microscopy with AGMK, BS-C-1 and RK_{13} cell cultures, hemagglutinin production in Vero cells and direct hemadsorption in BHK-21 cells have seen limited use but appear to be adequate procedures for virus isolation.

RELATIVE SENSITIVITY OF CELL CULTURES FOR
VIRUS ISOLATION

In Tables 4-II and 4-III data are summarized concerning the relative sensitivities of AGMK compared with RK_{13} and Vero cells for isolation of virulent and attenuated rubella viruses from throat swab specimens. In these studies the standard AGMK isolation procedures described earlier were followed. The RK_{13} cell cultures were inoculated, incubated and maintained similarly but were carried through two serial subcultures. The two types of cultures were shown to be of at least equivalent sensitivity for detecting virulent virus. All of 15 positive throat swab specimens yielded virus in both cell systems. These data are in good agreement with those reported by Schmidt *et al* (12) who found in parallel tests that AGMK, RK_{13} and BS-C-1 cells were similarly sensitive for the detection of natural virus in throat washings. On the basis of our studies it is not possible to assess accurately the possibility that the RK_{13} cells might be slightly more sensitive for the detection of attenuated virus; the observation that 5 of the 21 specimens shown to contain virus were positive in RK_{13} cells but negative in AGMK suggested that this might be true for the HPV-77 virus. However, this observation was not borne out in the experience with specimens from HPV-

TABLE 4-II

COMPARATIVE SENSITIVITY OF CELL CULTURES FOR RUBELLA VIRUS ISOLATION: PRIMARY AFRICAN GREEN MONKEY KIDNEY AND CONTINUOUS RK_{13} RABBIT KIDNEY CELLS

Type of Virus	No Specimens Tested	No. Specimens Positive for Virus			
		Total	GMK pos. RK_{13} pos.	GMK neg. RK_{13} pos.	GMK pos. RK_{13} neg.
Virulent*	16	15	15	0	0
Attenuated†					
HPV-77	22	21	16	5	0
HPV-120	21	21	19	1	1
Total	59	57	50	6	1

* Throat swab specimens collected within 1-3 days after the onset of rash from recruits with natural rubella acquired at Fort Dix, New Jersey, 1963.

† Throat swab specimens collected from vaccinees during the period from 10 to 20 days after immunization.

TABLE 4-III

COMPARATIVE SENSITIVITY OF CELL CULTURES FOR RUBELLA
VIRUS ISOLATION: PRIMARY AND CONTINUOUS VERO GREEN
MONKEY KIDNEY CELL CULTURES

| Type of Virus | No. Specimens Tested | Total | No. Specimens Positive for Virus | | |
			AGMK pos. Vero pos.	AGMK pos. Vero neg.	AGMK neg. Vero pos.
Virulent	38*	14	11	3	0
Attenuated	35†	17	6	6	5
Total	73	31	17	9	5

* Thirty-four throat swab and four heparinized blood specimens collected from 5 to 25 days after intranasal inoculation of rubella virus.
† Thirty-five throat swab specimens collected from subjects 12 to 24 days after vaccination. Vaccines used included HPV-77 DE5, HPV-77 DK12 and Benoit C, D and E level preparations.

120 vaccinees; here an equal number of positives were obtained in each cell system. Thus viruses could be easily recovered in both RK₁₃ and AGMK. The additional subpassage required in RK₁₃ cultures to allow the cells to manifest readily recognizable CPE made the RK₁₃ system slower in detecting virus.

In the comparison involving Vero cells, cultures were inoculated with 34 throat swabs and four heparinized blood specimens collected from subjects infected with natural rubella virus. Using identical techniques the originally inoculated AGMK and Vero cultures were incubated and maintained at 35°C for 10 days. Both types of cells were then subcultured in AGMK cells. No CPE was observed in Vero cultures. Eleven throat swabs yielded virus in both types of cultures. One swab specimen and two heparinized bloods were positive only in AGMK. It is apparent that specimens containing the attenuated virus were positive in AGMK alone or in Vero alone as often as they were shown to contain virus in both cell systems. It seems likely that this is the result of the very small amounts of virus present in these specimens (see Table 4-VII). The findings fail to confirm those reported earlier by Liebhaber *et al* (4) who suggested that Vero cells were 4.5 times more sensitive than GMK for primary virus isolation from the throat swabs and sera of infected chimpanzees. The discrepancy in results between these two studies might be explained by differences in Vero cell lines, since cells propagated in our laboratory also failed to show CPE with any rubella virus preparation even after attempts to adapt viruses by 14 serial subcultures. Alternatively the differences could be the result of a less sensitive lot of AGMK cells employed in the earlier study (see below). For whatever reason, in our experience Vero and AGMK cultures appeared to be of approximately equal sensitivity.

VARIATIONS IN SENSITIVITY OF SYSTEMS FOR DETECTION OF RUBELLA VIRUS

The systems employed for rubella virus isolation have shown a considerable variability from one laboratory to the next. For documentation of this, one needs only to compare the ability of various investigators to detect virus shedding in vaccinated children. For the same vaccine, rates ranging from 0% to 80% have been reported (26-28). Such variations may not be entirely related to cell culture; differing techniques of specimen collection, storage and inoculation may also contribute. For example, the addition of serum or bovine albumin to collection media stabilized the virus against thermal inactivation (1). Exposure to light resulted in rapid loss in infectivity of preparations stored in clear glass vials.

Ability to recover rubella virus was also strongly influenced by the status of the cell cultures employed. AGMK cultures may vary in sensitivity depending on the type of cell growth and the presence of extraneous agents. Experience has shown that poorly sheeted, granular AGMK monolayers frequently are unsuitable for detection of virus. Contamination of AGMK cultures with extraneous viruses may adversely affect their sensitivity. Cultures contaminated with SV-5 virus completely interfered with the growth of a 100 $TCID_{50}$ rubella virus inoculum, but failed to interfere significantly with the echovirus 11 challenge. SV-40 contaminated cultures, inoculated with rubella virus in the period before vacuolating CPE became apparent, similarly resisted rubella virus infection. Contamination with small amounts of foamy or simian cytomegaloviruses did not appear to affect adversely the sensitivity of cells for rubella virus.

Specific examples of variation in results obtained with continuous cell lines are also common. Schmidt and Lennette found BS-C-1 cells to be equivalent to AGMK cells for virus titration and noted that in cultures receiving limiting dilutions of virus, interference developed within seven days (12). In our experience, while these cells were sensitive for determination of virus infectivity, incubation for 15 days was required (9). Similarly, the behavior of cells used in cytopathic systems has occasionally been erratic. The amount of CPE which develops and the usefulness of the cell culture as a primary detection system has varied between laboratories. For example, Vero cells were reported to develop pronounced CPE with high passage levels of Mag and HPV-77 rubella virus strains (4, 13). Vero cultures derived from cells sent to us from Dr. Rhim (13), after passage in our laboratory, failed to show recognizable CPE with HPV-77 virus even after this strain had been serially subcultured 14 times in attempts to produce adaptation. Subculture of supernatant fluids from infected Vero cells to AGMK, however, demonstrated propagation of virus to high titer. The RK_{13} cell line may show a considerable degree of variation in the rate at which rubella CPE develops. In our laboratory, two morphologically similar lines of RK_{13} cells (both mycoplasma free) derived from the same parent culture have markedly different sensitivity for detecting rubella virus. These differences were reflected in the rapidity with which CPE developed. Thus, the type of cell culture employed cannot guarantee against the problems encountered in cell culture sensitivity. In our current practice the sensitivity of cultures used is monitored by assay of a reference preparation of known titer in each lot of cells. Titration values falling more than $0.5 \log_{10}$ units away from the geometric mean value are taken as an indication of the insensitivity of the cell lot and work performed in these lots is repeated.

PRESENCE OF VIRUS IN CLINICAL SPECIMENS

The virologic events attending virulent rubella virus infections have been well described (29, 30). Virus recovery data reported here were derived from the study of clinical specimens collected during epidemics of natural rubella at the Arkansas Children's

Colony. Virus isolation attempts were performed using the AGMK-echovirus type 11 interference technique. The results of isolation studies on serially collected specimens of blood from 11 subjects and daily throat swabs from 14 children are shown in Table 4-IV. During this epidemic, susceptible children who became infected showed from 1 to 4 positive blood specimens and from 9 to 28 positive pharyngeal specimens. Virus was readily recovered from the blood specimens of persons with rubella during the nine days preceding the appearance of rash; 27 of 33 viremia specimens were positive for virus. The appearance of the exanthem heralded the disappearance of circulating virus; viremia was seldom found later than the first day of rash. The disappearance of viremia appeared to coincide with the development of detectable neutralizing antibody. Pharyngeal swab specimens taken throughout the prodromal period were also frequently positive, and during the period from 5 days before until 4 days after rash, 95 to 96 percent of samples contained virus. A decreasing number of specimens continued to be positive for as long as three weeks following the onset of rash. Virus isolations beyond this period have been rare.

Pharyngeal excretion of virus also occurred in 80 to 92 percent of persons receiving attenuated vaccines; here, however, secretions were ordinarily positive for an average interval ranging from 3.5 to 4.8 days (31). The frequency with which throat swabs

TABLE 4-IV

FREQUENCY OF DEMONSTRABLE VIRUS IN HEPARINIZED BLOOD
AND PHARYNGEAL SWAB SPECIMENS COLLECTED FROM
CHILDREN WITH NATURAL RUBELLA

Day of Specimen Collection in Relation to Rash	Viremia Specimens		Pharyngeal Swab Specimens	
	No. Tested	% Positive for Virus	No. Tested	% Positive for Virus
–12 to 10	3	0	10	0
–9 to 6	12	67	41	42
–5 to 0	21	91	65	95
+1 to 4	11	36	53	96
+5 to 9	3	0	59	61
+10 to 14	0	—	57	35
+15 to 19	0	—	54	11
+20 to 21	0	—	16	13

TABLE 4-V

FREQUENCY OF DEMONSTRABLE PHARYNGEAL VIRUS SHEDDING
FOLLOWING RUBELLA IMMUNIZATION

Day After Vaccination	HPV-77 DE5 No. Tested	% Positive	HPV-77 DK12 No. Tested	% Positive	Cendehill No. Tested	% Positive
0-4	11	0	12	0	0	—
5-9	34	0	47	6	99	5
10-14	54	26	59	44	98	29
15-19	49	43	56	36	97	21
20-24	51	6	58	5	99	2
25-29	39	5	48	2	79	3

were positive during the period after vaccination with duck embryo and dog kidney derivatives of HPV-77 and the Cendehill rabbit kidney produced vaccine is indicated in Table 4-V. In each group less than 50 percent of specimens were positive during any interval studied. With each vaccine the highest frequency of virus recovery was observed from the tenth to the twentieth day after vaccination.

More virus was shed in the pharyngeal secretions of persons with natural disease than from vaccinees (Table 4-VI). Throat swab specimens from naturally infected and vaccinated persons were titrated in AGMK cultures. Geometric mean virus titers of specimens collected from persons with the natural disease were a hundredfold higher than those found in samples from vaccinees.

These data provide an explanation for the observation that virus was more readily and reproducibly detected in specimens

TABLE 4-VI

PHARYNGEAL EXCRETION OF VIRUS IN VIRULENT AND
ATTENUATED RUBELLA INFECTIONS

Type of Infection	No. Specimens Tested	Infectivity Titer $log_{10}/0.1$ ml Range	GMT*
Natural rubella	12†	0.5-3.8	2.4
HPV-77 vaccine	22‡	0.0-2.2	0.4

* GMT = Geometric mean titer
† Collected from 1 and 2 days before the onset of rash (5 swabs) on the day of rash (5 swabs) and on the 1st and 5th days after rash (1 swab each).
‡ Specimens collected from the 10th to 20th days after vaccination.

from subjects infected with natural rubella than from those from vaccinated persons. Other materials collected from persons infected with natural or attenuated viruses including stool (29), swabs of the uterine cervix (32) and joint effusion specimens were infrequently positive. Swabs of the uterine cervix were shown to be positive in three of six vaccinated pregnant women scheduled for therapeutic abortion. In 14 nonpregnant nursing students studied, only one of 27 serially collected cervical swabs yielded virus.

RECOVERY OF VIRUS IN MATERNAL-FETAL INFECTION

The ability to recover rubella virus during the major rubella epidemic which occurred in this country in 1964 added greatly to the fund of knowledge about congenital rubella infection and the rubella syndrome. Transmission of infection from mother to fetus was readily demonstrated (34-36). Virus was found in 30 percent and in 61 percent respectively of fetal and placental tissue suspensions prepared after therapeutic abortion for rubella (37). Virus was widely distributed in the tissues of infected fetuses. Data is presented in Table 4-VII concerning titration of rubella virus present in the tissues of an infected fetus studied in our laboratory. Therapeutic abortion was performed 57 days after the mother's rash appeared. Infectivity titers of several fetal organs and tissues ranged from $10^{2.5}$ to $10^{4.5}/1.0$ ml of 10% tissue suspension. Rawls *et al* (38) reported that virus recovery attempts were more often successful when cell cultures prepared from the fetal tissues were tested for virus than when tissue suspensions were assayed directly in AGMK cell cultures.

TABLE 4-VII

RUBELLA VIRUS INFECTIVITY TITERS OF FETAL TISSUES

Fetal Tissue	Infectivity Titer/1.0 ml of 10% Tissue Suspension
Face and eye	3.8
Mandible	3.5
Rib cage	3.5
Extremities (foot and hand)	3.1
Intestine	4.5
Liver	2.5
Placenta	1.6

TABLE 4-VIII

LABORATORY MARKERS OF RUBELLA VIRUS ATTENUTION

	Virus Characteristics	
Marker Test	*Virulent*	*Attenuated*
In vitro		
RK₁₃ CPE	Minimal at 35°C	Prompt, complete at 35°C
RK₁₃ plaques	Small, appear late	Large, appear early
Interferon induction	None or low levels	High levels
In vivo (rhesus monkeys)		
Virus shedding	More than 90%; sustained	Rarely observed; single episode when present
Viremia	Present in 50%	Not observed
Communicability	Frequent	Not observed
Antibody response (GMT)		
Neutralizing	High	Low
HI	High	Low
CF	High	Low or absent
Tissue dissemination and multiplication	Reticuloendothelial and many other tissues positive	Positive only in reticulo-endothelial system tissues
Intranasal infectivity	High; equal to tissue culture infectivity	Low; 100-fold less than tissue culture infectivity

Virus was also found to persist in the postnatal period. In fatal cases occurring in the first months of life, numerous organs were positive for virus indicating a widespread dissemination of the infection; virus shedding was also detected in throat, urine and fecal specimens (39, 40). Studies indicated that at birth approximately 80 percent of babies with congenital rubella excrete virus. This percentage gradually diminishes during the first year of life; by 15 months of age approximately 7 to 20 percent still excrete virus, and at 18 months only 5 percent still have positive specimens (41, 42). A recent report suggests that cultures of leukocytes from such children may also yield virus with some regularity during the first year of life (43).

MARKER TEST TECHNIQUES

The marker procedures developed in our laboratory to characterize rubella viruses are outlined in Table 4-VIII and have been reported in detail earlier (44). The three major procedures include tests for the ability of viruses to produce CPE and plaques in RK₁₃ cells, the interferon induction marker, and the marker dealing with the various characteristics of the infections produced in rhesus monkeys. Such procedures can be of assistance in differentiating between virulent and attenuated viruses.

DISCUSSION

A period of remarkable progress in our knowledge of rubella virus and rubella followed as a natural consequence of the isolation of the etiologic agent in 1962. Since the initial discovery, many cell culture systems have been devised for virus isolation and quantitation, although the AGMK-enterovirus challenge system continues to be widely used. Primary cultures have several advantages for virus isolation attempts; they (1) hold up well when inoculated with a variety of potentially noxious specimens; (2) exhibit early and complete interference with many cytopathic viruses; (3) show a reasonably constant cell composition, unaffected by the selective pressures of repeated serial passage; and (4) are available in most virus laboratories in this country. The disadvantage of the presence of contaminating extraneous agents in certain cell lots may however, necessitate repeat testing. In our experience with 64 lots of AGMK cells over the past 20 months, on only two occasions has repeat testing been required. Continuous cell lines such as Vero and RK₁₃ are equally sensitive, however, and have the theoretical advantage of freedom from extraneous agents. Cytopathic effects, however, may be variable with unadapted freshly isolated viruses and additional subcultures or subpassage to AGMK may be necessary to confirm the presence of rubella virus. With either system the importance of monitoring cell sensitivity with a continuing series of reference virus titrations cannot be overemphasized.

Virus isolation methods may be of assistance in the diagnosis of rubella. Since virus is regularly present in respiratory secretions and blood during the prodromal phase of illness, detection of virus may be accomplished by early convalescence. Also, virus may continue to be present in pharyngeal specimens for several weeks after antibodies have made their appearance. Thus isolation of virus may on occasion establish the diagnosis in subjects whose sera, obtained late, show high unchanging levels of rubella antibody. Recovery of virus may be helpful in the diagnosis of congenital rubella and may be a simpler first step than the detailed serum fractionation or immunofluorescent studies otherwise necessary. In the study of fetal tissues obtained at abortion the presence of virus in the cervical secretions must be sought; contamination of fetal tissues with maternal virus may be misleading. In congenitally infected infants, virus isolation may be of assistance in determining the period during which virus shedding and the risk of communicability occurs. Finally, the identification of virus isolates and the use of marker test techniques may be important when women are inadvertently immunized during pregnancy. Under such circumstances, the theoretical risk of transmission of attenuated virus to the fetus (32) makes consideration of therapeutic abortion necessary. Such unfortunate instances can provide invaluable additional information on this important question if careful virus isolation studies are performed.

SUMMARY

Rubella virus propagates in a variety of cell cultures and is most commonly recognized by the interference which it induces with the growth of other viruses. In several cell lines, especially those of rabbit origin, a marked cytopathic effect is produced. The ease with which rubella virus can be isolated during the prodromal phase of acute illness makes this procedure an important diagnostic tool.

REFERENCES

1. Weller, T. H., and Neva, F. A.: Propagation in tissue culture of cytopathic agents from patients with rubella-like illness. *Proc. Soc. Exp. Biol. Med.*, 111:215-225, 1962.
2. Parkman, P. D., *et al:* Recovery of rubella virus from army recruits. *Proc. Soc. Exp. Biol. Med.*, 111:225-230, 1962.
3. Hopps, H. E., *et al:* Biological characteristics of a continuous kidney cell line derived from the African Green monkey. *J. Immunol.*, 91:416-424, 1963.
4. Liebhaber, H., Riordan, J. T., and Horstmann, D. M.: Replication of rubella virus in a continuous line of African Green monkey kidney cells (Vero). *Proc. Soc. Exp. Biol. Med.*, 125:636-643, 1967.
5. Hull, R. N., Cherry, W. R., and Tritch, O. J.: Growth characteristics of monkey kidney cell strains LLC-MK$_1$, LLC-MK$_2$ and LLC-MK$_2$

(NCTC-3196) and their utility in virus research. *J. Exp. Med.*, 115:903-918, 1962.

6. McCarthy, K. G., Taylor-Robinson, C. H., and Pillinger, S. E.: Isolation of rubella virus from cases in Britain. *Lancet*, 2:593-598, 1963.

7. Stoker, M., and Macpherson, I.: Syrian hamster fibroblast cell line BHK-21 and its derivatives. *Nature*, 203:1355-1357, 1964.

8. Lennette, E. H., and Schmidt, N. J. (Eds.): Diagnostic Procedures for Viral and Rickettsial Diseases, 3rd ed., New York, American Public Health Association, Inc., 1964, p. 48.

9. Parkman, P. D., *et al:* Studies of rubella: I. Properties of the virus, *J. Immunol.*, 93:595-607, 1964.

10. Plotkin, S. A., Boue, A., and Boue, J. G.: The *in vitro* growth of rubella virus in human embryo cells. *Amer. J. Epidemiol.*, 81:71-85, 1965.

11. Veronelli, J. A., Maassab, H. F., and Hennessy, A. V.: Isolation in tissue culture of an interfering agent from patients with rubella. *Proc. Soc. Exp. Biol. Med.*, 111:472-476, 1962.

12. Schmidt, N. J., *et al:* Identification of rubella virus isolates by immufluorescent staining and a comparison of the sensitivity of three cell culture systems for recovery of virus. *J. Lab. Clin. Med.*, 68:502-509, 1966.

13. Rhim, J. S., and Schell, K.: Cytopathic and plaque assay of rubella virus in a line of African Green monkey kidney cells (Vero). *Proc. Soc. Exp. Biol. Med.*, 125:602-606, 1967.

14. Gunalp, A.: Growth and cytopathic effect of rubella virus in a line of Green monkey kidney cells. *Proc. Soc. Exp. Biol. Med.*, 118:85-90, 1965.

15. Desmyter, J., Melnick, J. L., and Rawls, W. E.: Defectiveness of interferon production and rubella virus interference in a line of African Green monkey kidney cells (Vero). *J. Virol.*, 2:955-961, 1968.

16. McCarthy, K., and Taylor-Robinson, C. H.: Growth and cytopathic effects of rubella virus in primary rabbit tissue culture. *Arch. Gesamte Virusforsch.*, 16:415-418, 1965.

17. Leirhay, J.: Cytopathic effect of rubella virus in a rabbit-cornea cell line. *Science*, 149:633-634, 1965.

18. Hull, R. N., and Butorac, G.: The utility of rabbit kidney cell strain, LLC-RK$_1$, to rubella virus studies. *Am. J. Epidemiol.*, 83:509-517, 1966.

19. Vaheri, A., *et al:* Cytopathic effect of rubella virus in BHK-21 cells and growth to high titers in suspension culture. *Virology*, 27:239-241, 1965.

20. Buynak, E. B., *et al:* Preparation and testing of duck embryo cell culture rubella vaccine. *Am. J. Dis. Child.*, 118:347-354, 1969.

21. Musser, S. J., and Hilsabeck, L. J.: Production of rubella virus vaccine, *Am. J. Dis. Child.*, 118:355-361, 1969.

22. Huygelen, C., *et al:* Safety testing of rubella virus vaccine (Cendehill strain). *Am. J. Dis. Child.,* 118:362-366, 1969.
23. Tint, H., and Rosanoff, E. I.: Production and testing of rubella virus vaccine. *Am. J. Dis. Child.,* 118:367-371, 1969.
24. Rafakjo, R. R.: In Proceedings of the International Conference of Rubella Immunization 1969. *Am. J. Dis. Child.,* 118:149-150, 1969.
25. Perlino, C. A., and Isacson, P.: Direct hemadsorption by cell cultures infected with rubella virus. *Am. J. Dis. Child.,* 118:83-84, 1969.
26. Stokes, J., Jr.: Discussion. In First International Conference on Vaccines Against Viral and Rickettsial Diseases of Man. Scientific Publication 147, Washington, D. C.: Pan American Health Organization and WHO, p. 402, 1967.
27. Martin du Pan, R., *et al:* Attenuation of rubella virus by serial passage in primary rabbit kidney cells. III. Clinical trial in infants. *Pediatr. Res.,* 2:38-42, 1968.
28. Meyer, H. M., Jr., Parkman, P. D., and Hopps, H. E.: The control of rubella. *Pediatrics,* 44:5-23, 1969.
29. Green, R. H., *et al:* Studies on the experimental transmission, clinical course, epidemiology and prevention of rubella. *Trans. Assoc. Am. Physicians,* 77:118-125, 1964.
30. Meyer, H. M., Jr., *et al:* Clinical studies with experimental live rubella virus vaccine (strain HPV-77) and evaluation of vaccine-induced immunity. *Am. J. Dis. Child.,* 115:648-654, 1968.
31. Meyer, H. M., Jr., *et al:* Attenuated rubella viruses. *Am. J. Dis. Child.,* 118:155-164, 1969.
32. Vaheri, A., *et al:* Transmission of attenuated rubella vaccines to the human fetus. *Am. J. Dis. Child.,* 118:243-246, 1969.
33. Stokes, J., *et al:* Vaccination of adult females with HPV-77 rubella vaccines. In *Proceedings of the 23rd Symposium on Microbiological Standardization: Rubella Vaccines* (London, November 1968). Basel, Switzerland, S. Karger, 1969.
34. Selzer, G.: Virus isolation, inclusion bodies and chromosomes in a rubella-infected human embryo. *Lancet,* 2:336-337, 1963.
35. Kay, H. E. M., *et al:* Congenital rubella infection of a human embryo.
36. Heggie, A. D., and Weir, W. C.: Isolation of rubella virus from a mother and fetus. *Pediatrics,* 34:278-280, 1964.
    Br. Med. J., 5042:166-167, 1964.
37. Weller, T. H., Alford, C. A., Jr., and Neva, F. A.: Changing epidemiologic concepts of rubella. *Yale J. Biol. Med.,* 37:455-467, 1965.
38. Rawls, W. E., *et al:* Spontaneous virus carrier cultures and postmortem isolation of virus from infants with congenital rubella. *Proc. Soc. Exp. Biol. Med.,* 120:623-626, 1965.
39. Monif, G. R., *et al:* Postmortem isolation of rubella virus from three children with rubella syndrome defects. *Lancet,* 1:723-724, 1965.

40. Bellanti, J. A., *et al:* Congenital rubella. *Am. J. Dis. Child.*, 110:464-472, 1965.
41. Cooper, L. Z., and Krugman, S.: Diagnosis and management: congenital rubella. *Pediatrics,* 37:335-338, 1966.
42. Rawls, W. E., *et al:* Persistent virus infection in congenital rubella. *Arch. Ophthalmol.* 77:430-433, 1967.
43. Jack, I., and Grutzner, J.: Cellular viremia in babies infected with rubella virus before birth. *Br. Med. J.*, 1:289-292, 1969.
44. Hopps, H. E., Parkman, P. D., and Meyer, H. M., Jr.: Laboratory testing in rubella vaccine control. *Am. J. Dis. Child.*, 118:338-346, 1969.

Chapter 5

DIAGNOSTIC PROCEDURES IN A CLINICAL LABORATORY

GILBERT M. SCHIFF and THOMAS ROTTE

INTRODUCTION

THE laboratory of the Clinical Virology Section (CVS) of the College of Medicine, University of Cincinnati, was established five and a half years ago. During this time the laboratory has been engaged in many facets of rubella research. In addition, the CVS has provided rubella diagnostic services for the medical community, and recently has been involved in the establishment of a program designed to achieve control of rubella infection in our community. The program involves the use of the laboratory to confirm the diagnosis of acquired and congenital rubella, to determine the immune status of childbearing-age females, to identify susceptible pregnant women for close surveillance and consideration for administration of immune globulin (IG), and to utilize rubella vaccines intelligently. The purpose of this presentation is to describe the role and functions of the diagnostic laboratory in this type of control program.

RUBELLA CONTROL ASSISTANCE

The availability of laboratory tests to document active rubella infection and to identify the susceptible childbearing-age woman is crucial to any control program. The CVS has provided laboratory confirmation of the clinical diagnosis of rubella (see Table 5-I). The inadequacy of clinical diagnosis alone in cases of suspected rubella infection is all too familiar and can lead to tragic events if a pregnancy is involved. There have been many false-positive and false-negative clinical diagnoses of rubella. Many viruses which cause rubella-like clinical illnesses lack the teratogenic potential of the rubella virus. I wonder how many non-rubella infections have been responsible for needless termination

51

TABLE 5-I

CLINICAL VIROLOGY SECTION: RUBELLA CONTROL ASSISTANCE

1. Diagnosis of active disease
   a. Acquired infection
   b. Congenital infection
2. Identification of susceptibles
   a. Pregnant women
   b. All childbearing-age females
   c. Age-group susceptibility rates
3. Vaccine assistance
   a. Closed population studies
   b. Family studies
   c. School-age programs
   d. Consultative services

of pregnancy and have caused many months of mental anguish by the expectant woman and her family.

Misdiagnosis can result in other types of problems. We recently conducted a city-wide rubella vaccine evaluation in Dayton, Ohio schools which was followed by a large-scale outbreak of erythema infectiosa in a nearby community. In addition to many nonvaccinated children with rash disease, there were several adults with rash followed by arthralgia and arthritis. Laboratory study ruled out rubella, but only after false implication of the vaccine.

On the other hand, rubella frequently is atypical or subclinical and is often not even considered in the diagnosis. This situation also has obvious serious implications. Our laboratory has assisted in the diagnosis of congenital rubella. The diagnosis of congenital rubella infection can be confirmed in the laboratory by viral isolation and serological tests. The diagnosis can also be made retrospectively. During the 1964-1965 epidemic, the CVS undertook a massive screening program on all newborns at the Cincinnati General Hospital to define the incidence of congenital rubella infection. The findings suggested that a significant amount of intra-uterine rubella infection was unsuspected and would have been missed if laboratory tests had not been used. While it is presently impractical to test all newborns, certainly suspected cases should be tested. Identification of the congenital rubella infants who are positive shedders of virus is important to control the spread of infection. All infants so identified by us have been followed serially to determine when rubella virus shedding ceases.

We have determined the immune status of several female populations, which has aided or will aid in their future management against rubella infection. The identification of childbearing-age susceptibles, especially pregnant women before they become exposed, makes it possible to accurately diagnose rubella infection upon exposure. It also makes possible the consideration of the prophylactic administration of immune globulin in pregnant women. The use of immune globulin against rubella infection in pregnancy is controversial. The conflicting results of the past probably reflect the interaction of several factors: unknown immune status of the recipients, lack of confirmatory laboratory diagnosis, variation in dose and titer of the immune globulin, and variation in the time of administration of IG in relation to time of exposure. Recent studies from our laboratory indicated that administration of high-titered IG within twenty-four hours of the intranasal instillation of a rubella challenge virus in adults prevented the expected viremia and infection. There was also some evidence that prophylactic administration of IG was effective. However, a recent study by Cooper *et al* in children failed to show prevention of infection. They have not determined the effect on viremia as yet. At any rate, it is our belief that in cases of susceptible pregnant women exposed to rubella who would not consider termination of pregnancy, IG should be given in hopes of some positive effect.

Routine immune testing of childbearing-age (postmenarchial) females will permit selective, careful vaccination of these women. We have negotiated with several high school districts to institute routine testing of senior females. From studies performed in the area high schools, we have shown that acquisition of rubella immunity in the high school period during inter-epidemic years was negligible. Since these are the females who soon will be bearing children, vaccination appears indicated. Of course, the problem of pregnancy in high school must still be considered. Establishment of routine immune testing of childbearing-age females will also serve as a safety check on the persistence of artificial immunity in children receiving vaccination many years previously.

Our laboratory is assisting in the community use of rubella vaccines. In the last two years we have vaccinated several populations as part of the national vaccine evaluation program. Based on this experience, the community is approaching vaccination of prepubertal children in two ways—first, the immediate mass vaccination of school-age children in the schools. This will be accompanied by the administration of vaccine to pre-school-age children in public health clinics and private offices. After this "crash" program, routine vaccination of children will occur through the clinics and private physicians. Vaccination of postpubertal women is being recommended on an individual basis only after a prevaccination blood test demonstrates need for vaccination, and pregnancy can be ruled out at the time of vaccination and for eight weeks afterwards. Postvaccination antibody titers on the postpubertal vaccinees are also recommended and offered. In this conjunction, the CVS has agreed to do prevaccination and postvaccination blood tests on adult women. We also have agreed to train personnel from hospital and commercial laboratories in the test methods. Another role that the diagnostic lab can assume in support of vaccination programs is to provide the crucial, necessary long-term surveillance on the vaccinees to determine protection afforded during subsequent natural rubella challenge situations.

LABORATORY FACILITIES

The CVS has had the advantage of several years' experience with the diagnostic procedures employed for rubella in conjunction with a large research effort. The demand to provide diagnostic services has led us to set up a diagnostic unit, which I will describe. We use two laboratories. One laboratory is used for viral isolation and neutralization tests. The other laboratory is for HI and CF tests. Three technicians are involved. One is responsible for rubella viral isolation and identification and neutralization tests. A second technician handles the HI testing on a full-time basis. She is assisted by a third technician who also performs the CF testing. Patients are encouraged to come to the laboratories for collection of specimens and histories. We attempt to complete and report all HI and CF tests within five days of obtaining the specimen. Perhaps our largest headache occurs in the record-keeping and reporting department. Reports are sent to both the referring physician and the patient, and this requires a part-time secretary. During an average week, up to 70 tests are performed. Recently this work load has increased.

Rubella isolation and identification are performed by the interference technique, utilizing primary African green monkey kidney (AGMK) tissue cultures, Coxsackie A-9 superinfection, and ferret hyperimmune sera. Three passages are performed before a specimen is considered negative. Control positive rubella virus is titrated in each lot of AGMK tissue to determine tissue sensitivity. Tissue cultures are purchased. We have used other viral detection systems, such as Vero cells, RK-13, and Sirc cell plaque assay. In our hands, the interference system is more sensitive in isolating viruses from raw specimens. Viral isolation is attempted on all suspected rubella patients with rash, including contacts to whom the patients are exposed, and on infants with congenital infection. In the latter patients, serial isolation efforts are made to monitor duration of viral shedding. We attempt to isolate virus from the suspected contact or vector who has exposed the pregnant patient because we have found that follow-up collection of blood specimens from the contacts is often not accomplished, making serological diagnosis difficult.

The serological tests performed by our laboratory include HI, CF, and neutralization antibody tests. Since the development of the HI test, we have not performed many neutralization tests. We have set up the FA test system but do not use it routinely. The bulk of our testing involves the HI test. The test system employed is essentially that of Stewart *et al*, using 4 units of antigen; a 4+ end point; kaolin and adult chick cell adsorption; one-day-old chick rbc's in Alsevers; and microtiter equipment. The antigen is purchased from Flow Laboratories. Each test run includes positive and negative human and ferret sera and antigen titrations. Patients' sera are tested for nonspecific agglutination and are tested in duplicate on separate test days. Paired specimens are tested on all exposed pregnant women unless the situation permits an accurate interpretation on a single specimen. The HI test is used to make a serological diagnosis of active rubella and to determine rubella immune status. In situations where blood specimens are taken relatively late in the course of illness and retrospective diagnosis is required, HI testing is supplemented with mercaptoethanol treatment and CF tests. The CF antibody test employed is that of Sever *et al,* using 2 units of antigen, 2 exact units of complement, and microtiter equipment. The CF antigen is purchased. Test specimens are run as pairs and in duplicate.

Recently, we have compared our HI test system with the system developed by Liebhaber, which substitutes dextran sulfate and calcium adsorption for kaolin, and utilizes goose cells. We are impressed with the relative ease of the test and the sharpness of end points. We are seriously considering conversion to the D-S-C system.

In our laboratory an HI titer of 16 or greater is associated with immunity, while a titer of < 8 means susceptibility. A titer of 8 is borderline, although it usually means immunity as determined by human volunteer challenge studies. Comparison of HI antibody titers found in our laboratory to those of other laboratories is consistent, although we have a tendency to be one or two dilutions lower when antibody titer is present.

PROBLEMS ASSOCIATED WITH SEROLOGICAL TESTS

We have encountered several problems in the performance of these tests. There have been variations in the titer of the HI antigen despite identical lot pedigree. This has resulted in the use of higher or lower concentrations of antigen than desired. Reproducibility of HI test results is about 95 percent, requiring duplication of testing of all "important" specimens. Tissue culture sensitivity to rubella virus varies considerably, so that proper controls to determine degree of sensitivity is mandatory.

A frequent situation that the diagnostic laboratory faces is that of the pregnant woman exposed to a child with a rash diagnosed clinically as rubella. The laboratory is called on to make or rule out a diagnosis of rubella in the woman. The way that we handle this situation is the following:

1. An "acute" blood is obtained from the woman for HI and possible CF tests. We recommend the administration of IG as soon as possible if exposure has not been over 6 days and the woman agrees to be followed with serial HI tests.

2. The child is sought to obtain throat swabs and paired blood specimens for diagnostic tests. Although the diagnosis will take several weeks, a positive diagnosis makes it imperative to follow the woman carefully and to search for other exposed people.

3. Serial bloods are collected from the woman for HI and possible CF tests. It has been our experience that the IG administration does not interfere with the serological diagnosis.

COMMENTS AND SUMMARY

The CVS laboratory has had several years' experience in providing rubella diagnostic services to the community. We have frequently aided the clinician in the management of difficult situations. To my knowledge, we have yet to err in the proper determination of immune status or in missing clinical or subclinical rubella (whether or not IG was administered) which resulted in the birth of a defective infant. We also have encountered situations in which retrospective diagnosis of acquired or congenital rubella was not possible. With the advent of mass rubella vaccination programs, the role of the diagnostic laboratory will be even more significant.

Chapter 6

CONTROL OF LABORATORY TESTS FOR RUBELLA AT THE STATE LEVEL

Jay E. Satz

IN discussing the role of the state public health laboratory in the diagnosis of rubella infections it is first necessary to briefly describe the major responsibilities of the state laboratory to public health. The following description may not apply to all state laboratories for there are several parameters, such as size of population, geographic area and number of urban centers, which may limit a state public health laboratory's activity.

The first function of the state laboratory is to act as a reference center. This is to confirm the results of clinical laboratories. The state public health laboratory at one time was considered as a routine testing service for the community. However, in recent years this stereotyped image has changed because of the rapid progress which has taken place in the field of laboratory medicine. Patient diagnosis was once a major responsibility of the state public health laboratory, but in many states this activity has been limited to a reference function, unless a specific epidemiologic program is associated with this activity or a diagnostic procedure is too complex and economically unfeasible for smaller laboratories to perform.

The second function of the state laboratory is to recommend to local clinical laboratories new methodology and changes in older basic laboratory procedures. This can only be derived by a comparative investigation of these procedures. After determining by a thorough comparative study that a new procedure can be used, it is the responsibility of the state laboratory to help train personnel from clinical laboratories in the new technic. This can be accomplished by either having training on an individual basis or

---

From the Division of Laboratories, Pennsylvania Department of Health.

by holding training sessions for large groups of technical personnel. The latter has the advantage of rapidly training a larger number of individuals at one time.

A third responsibility of the state laboratory is to support epidemiological programs. This involves collaboration with field public health officers in studying communicable disease problems in the community. The laboratory may also aid in control of infectious diseases by testing immunological responses following the administration of new vaccines.

The fourth and final responsibility of many state health laboratories is the certification of clinical laboratories. This certification is dependent upon inspection of equipment and facilities of the laboratory and the demonstration of qualified personnel which is usually determined by proficiency evaluations. The latter is an extremely important index of the competence of a specific laboratory. Proficiency evaluations are also important in determining whether a new procedure can be effectively performed by these laboratories.

Since rubella infections during first trimester pregnancies frequently lead to congenital malformations, the accurate and early diagnosis of this disease has become of prime importance. Clinically this disease is difficult to diagnose accurately. Therefore, it is necessary to rely on laboratory tests for positive diagnosis. As in all viral infections, the laboratory diagnosis of rubella depends upon isolation of the agent from clinical specimens and/or the detection of developing specific antibody. Until recently, these tests were extremely difficult to perform because of the complexity of technics for propagating the virus and therefore, these tests were only carried out on a limited basis as a special diagnostic service by state and federal public health laboratories and occasionally by a research institution.

With the recent development of the rapid hemagglutination-inhibition test for rubella it is now possible that most clinical laboratories can aid in the diagnosis of rubella. The laboratory diagnosis of most virus infections has not usually benefited the patient because results are obtained too late and the patient has usually recovered. There is also no treatment for most of the virus diseases. Therefore, physicians will not usually consider that such costly tests are justified. However, in the case of rubella, particularly in women during the first or second trimester of pregnancy, rapid diagnosis is extremely important in order to ascertain if there is the possibility of fetal infection. Knowledge of the immunological status of the patient is also helpful to the physician because it is believed that the presence of antibodies in the mother's serum, due to a prior infection, will prevent infection of the fetus. Therefore, laboratory tests to determine either the possibility of a rubella infection or the immunological status of a patient can now be justified. This information can be extremely valuable in determining the course of action a physician must undertake when he is faced with the possibility of a rubella infection.

Since the hemagglutination-inhibition test has been found to be simple to perform and results are obtained in a matter of hours, the procedure lends itself to large-scale testing. A study was initiated by the Pennsylvania Department of Health to determine whether it would be practical to introduce a rubella testing system into routine clinical laboratories and to ascertain whether serious practical problems might exist in such a system.

One hospital and five independent laboratories located in the Philadelphia area were selected for the study. Representatives of each laboratory attended a one-day session at the facilities of the Pennsylvania Department of Health, Division of Laboratories, where they were given instruction in the rubella HI test using the microtechnique (1).

The training was performed by the personnel of the Pennsylvania Department of Health assisted by representatives of Flow Laboratories, Rockville, Maryland. All equipment and reagents were provided by Flow Laboratories and they had been previously tested by the Division of Laboratories for specificity, sensitivity and reproducibility. At the end of the training session, each representative was given a kit containing materials and reagents needed to perform the HI test. In addition, each laboratory was given the same 120 pretested sera for evaluation. The serum samples were prepared by our laboratories using pools of known positive and negative sera. Each laboratory was also asked to collect their own individual routine specimens, test them by the HI test and send aliquots of each to the Pennsylvania Department of Health, Division of Laboratories for confirmatory testing. All sera used in the evaluation were tested at dilutions of 1:10 and 1:20. Results of the tests were recorded as positive (inhibition of hemagglutination at 1:10 and/or 1:20), negative (no inhibition at 1:10) or nonspecific (serum control demonstrating hemagglutination).

Hemagglutination-inhibition tests were performed by the six laboratories on the same 120 serum samples. The results from 5 out of 6 laboratories showed a 100 percent correlation with the results from the state laboratory. The sixth laboratory missed 1 out of 120 serum samples. The results of the comparison between each of the independent laboratories and the Pennsylvania Department of Health Laboratory using their own routine serum specimens are presented in Table 6-I. Three out of the six laboratories demonstrated 100 percent agreement with our laboratory's results. The other three laboratories showed agreements of 97.5, 98, and 99 percent. The overall agreement between the six laboratories and our laboratory was 99 percent. Only 6 of the 691 sera tested showed disagreement.

In the case of the comparison between our laboratory and test laboratory number 2, there were two sera that showed disagreement. One serum was found to be positive by our laboratory and negative by the test laboratory, while the second serum was found to be negative by our laboratory and positive by the test laboratory.

Since the results of the preliminary rubella workshop suggested that routine clinical laboratories are capable of effectively performing the HI test, it was decided to offer workshops to all laboratories in the Commonwealth of Pennsylvania. Training sessions were set up in Philadelphia at the facilities of the Division of Laboratories, Pennsylvania Department of Health and in Pittsburgh at the facilities of the Allegheny County Health Department. Three one-day workshops were conducted in each city. Two hundred representatives from 152 private and hospital laboratories attended these sessions. Since the agents and procedures used for the preliminary training sessions were found to be ef-

TABLE 6-I

COMPARISON OF RESULTS BETWEEN THE LABORATORY OF THE PA. DEPARTMENT OF HEALTH AND SIX INDEPENDENT LABORATORIES IN THE PERFORMANCE OF THE HEMAGGLUTINATION-INHIBITION TEST FOR RUBELLA

Test	No. of Sera Tested*	Results of Test Lab			Results of State Lab			Disagreement Between Test & State Labs (No. of Sera)	Agreement Between Test & State Labs—%
		Pos.	Neg.	Non-spec.	Pos.	Neg.	Non-spec.		
1	124	117	7	0	117	7	0	0	100
2	105	87	16	2	87	16	2	2	98
3	96	90	4	1	90	4	1	0	100
4	120	110	9	1	110	9	1	0	100
5	120	109	5	6	109	7	4	3	97.5
6	124	117	7	0	118	6	0	1	99
Total	691							6	Overall Agreement 99%

* Each group of sera from the individual labs represents their own routine specimens from women of childbearing age.

fective, they were also used for the six workshops. Two companies, Flow Laboratories, Rockville, Maryland and Grand Island Biological Company, Grand Island, New York, assisted in the workshops and furnished the reagents needed to perform the tests.

Presently, in the Commonwealth of Pennsylvania there are at least 35 hospital and private laboratories performing the rubella HI test. The majority of these laboratories are located in the eastern and western sections of the state where they can service the majority of the population.

It seems evident from these observations that a rubella serologic testing system utilizing the hemagglutination-inhibition test can be established as a practical routine procedure in clinical laboratories. The test procedure was found to be easily handled by the participating laboratories and the results obtained on the comparative testing demonstrated that the HI test could be performed proficiently. It is interesting to note that the six clinical laboratories involved in the initial study were only given the one day of training and at no time during the comparison study which took several weeks did they need additional instruction.

The reliability of reagents is, however, a critical factor which was controlled in this study. It is conceivable that lack of consistency in commercial products could lead to erroneous results on a routine basis unless some mechanism is provided to approve or certify all lots of reagents.

With a large number of independent laboratories performing the hemagglutination-inhibition test the public has a more efficient diagnostic service at the community level. There is a greater tendency to utilize such services when they are available locally than if specimens must be shipped to a centralized facility. However, for this type of system to work effectively the state laboratory must provide a program where these laboratories are evaluated on a routine periodic basis in order to ascertain that optimum proficiency is maintained.

The Commonwealth of Pennsylvania has initiated such a program. It consists of periodically sending to laboratories unknown serum specimens for the determination of rubella hemagglutination-inhibition antibody titers. The same serum specimens are also sent to laboratories located outside the state which can act as reference centers. These are usually state and federal public health laboratories.

The first proficiency evaluation of laboratories in Pennsylvania performing the rubella hemagglutination-inhibition test was conducted in September of 1969. Eighty percent of these clinical laboratories passed the first evaluation. The results of this evaluation indicated that the main problem in the test was associated with the fact that there are several types of methods now being routinely employed for the detection of rubella HI antibodies. These included the micro and macro dilution technics and different methods recommended by several commercial companies. These methods not only differ in the mechanical performance of the test but also in the types of reagents used, such as buffers, red blood cells and antigen. Problems may arise if these reagents from different commercial sources are mixed. This can reduce both the specificity and sensitivity of the test. The results of our first evaluation has made it clear that proper control and standardization of the rubella HI test is necessary in order to offer the public a reliable diagnostic service.

The HI test for the detection of rubella antibodies can be an important procedure for aiding in the diagnosis of the disease, if properly applied. We have recommended that the test be performed either as a diagnostic procedure in which two serum samples (acute and convalescent) are needed or as a screening procedure to determine the rubella immunological status, particularly in women of childbearing age. For the latter purpose, it is not important to determine a rise in antibody level and therefore, the test can be performed at a limited number of low dilutions, such as 1:10 and 1:20. Sera which do not inhibit hemagglutination at a dilution of 1:10 should be considered as a possible negative, and the patient may be susceptible to rubella. Sera which only inhibit hemagglutination at 1:10 and not at 1:20 should be considered as questionable, since nonspecific inhibitors of hemagglutination have been detected at a 1:10 dilution of serum from some individuals even after treatment with kaolin. Sera which inhibit hemagglutination at both dilutions should be considered positive, and the patients are unlikely to contract rubella. This problem of removal on nonspecific inhibitors may be resolved in the near future by the treatment of sera with either manganous chloride-heparin or dextran sulfate $CaCl_2$ (2, 3). These preparations have been shown to be more efficient in the removal of these inhibitors than the normal kaolin treatment.

Since approximately 15 percent of women of childbearing age have no antibodies to rubella and therefore are susceptible to the disease, these individuals should be tested at appropriate intervals in order to detect a change in their immune status and also at any time that exposure to rubella is suspected. It is extremely important that women who were previously negative are tested at monthly intervals during the first five months of gestation, since this method of testing could detect an inapparent rubella infection. The test can also be applied to patients who are exposed to rubella in the first trimester of pregnancy. If the individual had not been previously tested, the presence of HI antibodies in such an early postexposure specimen provides evidence of immunity rather than evidence of infection.

This procedure can also be of value when associated with a rubella vaccine program. The physician will know, through the testing program, which females are susceptible to rubella and thus require immunization. Since the HI test has been shown to detect antibodies after infection with attenuated rubella virus, it can be used to determine the effectiveness of immunization.

Together with a large-scale clinical laboratory testing program utilizing the hemagglutination-inhibition test the state public health laboratory must provide additional rubella laboratory diagnostic services. This should include isolation of the virus from clinical specimens from patients suspected of having rubella. This is extremely useful for a diagnosis of rubella in newborns with congenital malformations. These infants with congenital rubella usually excrete virus for long periods of time after birth. Serological diagnosis in these cases is usually limited because of the presence of maternal antibody which persists for several months after birth. Isolation of the virus would also be helpful in cases where a differentiation must be made between infection due to either vaccine or wild virus strains.

Since serum samples are not always obtained at the proper

time intervals during a possible rubella infection, which limits the usefulness of the hemagglutination-inhibition test, other serological procedures such as the complement-fixation test (4) and the demonstration of rubella specific IgM antibody (2, 5, 6) should be offered by the state public health laboratory to ascertain if infection has occurred. The hemagglutination-inhibition test is useful as a diagnostic procedure only when it can measure an elevation in antibody level, thus two serum samples are needed from the patient. Frequently only a single serum specimen is obtained, usually after the appearance of clinical symptoms, and the presence of HI antibodies in this type of serum sample is not indicative of infection.

The complement-fixation test and the demonstration of rubella IgM antibody may be useful in determining recent rubella infections. The complement-fixation test has been proven valuable in establishing a diagnosis of actual disease because of the transient property of the CF antibodies. The CF response may occur several days or even weeks after the appearance of clinical symptoms and this antibody response usually decreases very rapidly (4). The presence of these antibodies in a single serum specimen particularly in high concentration may be indicative of a recent infection. Because this test has limited use as compared to the HI test and the preparation of reagents are costly, it is not adaptable for routine use in clinical laboratories. Therefore, the state public health laboratory should offer this service for cases of rubella where the other technics fail to make a definitive diagnosis.

The demonstration of rubella HI specific IgM antibody may also be useful in determining a recent infection because these antibodies have been found to be only present during the early phase of the disease, usually several days after the rash (2). These antibodies may be detected simply by treating sera with 2-mercaptoethanol, which is a sulphydryl reducing compound that inactivates IgM antibody. Therefore, a fourfold reduction in HI titer after treatment with this compound provides evidence of a recent rubella infection. However, this test is limited to only serum samples obtained from one to seven days after the appearance of the rash. After this time interval these IgM antibodies decrease rapidly being replaced by the normal IgG antibodies which are not sensitive to 2-mercaptoethanol treatment.

The demonstration of rubella specific IgM antibodies using sucrose-density gradient ultracentrifugation (5) or Sephadex gel filtration (6) may be useful in the serodiagnosis of congenital rubella. Since maternal antibodies are of the IgG type the demonstration of rubella specific IgM antibodies in newborn sera would be indicative of a fetal rubella infection. Since this method has limited use like the complement-fixation test it also should be offered by the state public health laboratory as a supplemental serodiagnostic procedure for rubella infections.

In conclusion the state public health laboratory can aid in the control of rubella by providing adequate rubella diagnostic services such as the following:

1. Training of laboratory personnel in the performance of the hemagglutination-inhibition test.

2. Evaluating laboratories in this test in order to ascertain that optimum proficiency is maintained.

3. Confirming serologic conversions or other test results.

4. Pretesting of all commercial rubella diagnostic reagents.

5. Offering other supplemental diagnostic procedures such as isolation of the virus, complement-fixation test and demonstration of rubella specific IgM antibodies.

REFERENCES

1. National Communicable Disease Center Laboratory Consultation and Development Section. Atlanta, Georgia, 1969. Modification of: Halonen, P. E., Ryan, J. M., and Stewart, J. A.: Rubella hemagglutinin prepared with alkaline extraction of virus grown in suspension culture of BHK-21 cells. *Proc. Soc. Exp. Biol. Med.*, 125:162-167, 1967.

2. Cooper, L. Z., Matters, B., Rosenblum, J. K., and Krugman, S.: Experience with a modified rubella hemagglutination-inhibition antibody test. *JAMA*, 207:89-93, 1969.

3. Liebhaber, H.: Removal of non-specific inhibitors from human sera with dextran sulfate and $CaCl_2$. Presented at Northeast Regional Conference on Rubella, 1969.

4. Sever, J. L., Hubner, R. J., Costellano, G. A., Sarma, P. S., Fabiyi, A., Schiff, G. M., and Cusumano, C. L.: Rubella complement-fixation test. *Science*, 148:385-387, 1965.

5. Alford, C. A., Jr.: Studies on antibody in congenital rubella infections. *Am. J. Dis. Child.*, 77:455-463, 1965.

6. Bellanti, J. A., Artenstein, M. S., Olson, L. C., Buescher, E. L., Luhrs, C. E., and Milstead K. L.: Congenital rubella. *Am. J. Dis. Child.*, 77:464-472, 1965.

Chapter 7

CONTROL OF RUBELLA LABORATORY TESTS AT THE FEDERAL LEVEL

Kenneth L. Herrmann

THERE is little doubt that the development of the rubella hemagglutination-inhibition (HI) technique (1, 2) has had a major impact on rubella testing in laboratories, big and small, throughout the United States. The availability of commercial reagents at reasonable cost has put this test within the reach of almost every clinical diagnostic laboratory. At the International Rubella Conference in Bethesda in February, 1969, it was stated that we are approaching the time when rubella immunity screening should be available to every woman of childbearing age. If one estimates that there are roughly 20 to 25 million women in that category, it may be quickly seen that we are far from reaching that idealistic goal at the present time. However, just four years ago less than one-fifth of our state health department laboratories were able to perform rubella diagnostic tests. Today, all but six state laboratories offer this testing service. The major reason for this increase is, without question, the availability of the rubella HI test.

With the licensure of an effective vaccine against rubella, laboratory diagnostic testing and immunity screening for this disease has assumed an increasingly important role. Although many more laboratories, both governmental and private, are now able to undertake rubella tests, there is growing concern over the reliability of these tests in some laboratories, especially those which would perform rubella tests on a small scale or infrequent basis.

From the U.S. Department of Health, Education, and Welfare, Public Health Service, Health Services and Mental Health Administration, National Communicable Disease Center, Atlanta, Georgia 30333.

Editor's Note: Recently a standardized procedure has been developed and recommended by the committee. Details are available from CDC.

The U.S. Public Health Service has made a goal to insure that accurate rubella diagnostic tests are available to all physicians. The efforts currently being directed at the federal level toward achieving this goal are the subject of my discussion today.

The U.S. Public Health Service is giving high priority to developing means and guidelines for upgrading the overall quality and reliability of rubella testing services. These efforts are primarily being channeled in three general areas of activity: (1) improvement and standardization of the rubella HI test procedure itself, (2) control of quality of reagents available, and (3) training.

As more and more laboratories have begun undertaking rubella HI testing, shortcomings in the performance of the test have become evident. At present, the HI test for rubella is not a standardized technique, and several modifications of the test are in use (1-6).* Comparison of results from different laboratories on the same serum specimens have shown widely variant results. Some of the numerous variables in the test according to the various procedure modifications include the buffer diluents used, pH of the reaction mixture, procedure for removal of nonspecific inhibitors and agglutinins, temperature of reaction, the type of indicator red blood cells used, and the procedure (macro vs. micro) recommended. The National Communicable Disease Center (Center for Disease Control) is presently collaborating with several other nationally recognized rubella virus laboratories* to assess these variables in the test and arrive at a standard recommended procedure. Such a standardized procedure would be of great help toward eliminating many of the pitfalls encountered with the HI test at present and would allow greater uniformity of reagent quality to be achieved.

Since rubella serology is performed primarily for two basically different purposes—the first being for determination of immunity status of an individual or a given population, and the second for

---

* Yale University School of Medicine (Dr. Dorothy M. Horstmann), New York University School of Medicine (Dr. Louis Z. Cooper), California State Department of Public Health (Dr. Edwin H. Lenette), University of Michigan School of Medicine (Dr. Joseph V. Baublis), and Columbia University School of Medicine (Dr. Paul D. Ellner).

diagnostic confirmation of a suspected rubella illness—it is of critical importance that the antibody test be able to accurately separate the seropositive from the seronegative individuals as well as distinguish between differences of antibody titer in paired sera. Sensitivity of the test system together with effectiveness of removal of nonspecific inhibitors are both of critical importance for accurate immunity screening. The intralaboratory test variability or reproducability has strong bearing on the accuracy of detecting significant changes of antibody levels indicative of recent rubella infection.

In the course of the collaborative study being coordinated by the NCDC, we have had an opportunity to examine the inter- and intralaboratory reproducibility and sensitivity of rubella HI tests carried out using a variety of different technical modifications as summarized in Table 7-I. Each of the six laboratories in this study received identical sets of 94 randomly coded specimens (47 duplicates) ranging from negative to high titer. Results revealed considerable interlaboratory variation of titers, emphasizing the hazard of comparing the results of one laboratory's testing with that of another. Table 7-II shows the relative accuracy of these six laboratories in distinguishing positive from negative rubella sera. Laboratory II, using one of the commercial kit procedures and reagents, had the greatest difficulty in detecting low level rubella antibody with a false-negative rate of 10.2 percent; while Laboratory III was found to have the greatest

TABLE 7-I

COLLABORATIVE RUBELLA HI STANDARDIZATION STUDY PROCEDURES USED FOR COMPARATIVE RUBELLA HI TEST EVALUATION

Lab #	Serum Treatment Method	pH	Buffer Diluent Sr. & An.	Cells	RBC's
I	Kaolin (pH 9)	9.0→6.2	BABS	PBS	Chick
II	Kaolin (pH 7)	7.2	DGV	DGV	Duracyte™
III-A	Heparin-MnCl₂	6.3	HSAG	HSAG	Goose
III-B	Dextran sulfate-CaCl₂	6.3	HSAG	HSAG	Goose
IV	Kaolin (pH 9)	9.0→6.2	BABS	PBS	Chick
V	Heparin-MnCl₂	7.2	DGV	DGV	Chick
VI	Heparin-MnCl₂	7.2	DGV	DGV	Chick

TABLE 7-II

COLLABORATIVE RUBELLA HI STANDARDIZATION STUDY
ANALYSIS OF FALSE-POSITIVE AND FALSE-NEGATIVE RESULTS

	I %	II %	III A %	III B %	IV %	V_1 %	V_2 %	VI %
				Laboratory No.				
False-Positive	0.0	0.0	43.8	18.8	0.0	3.1	0.0	6.2
False-Negative	2.6	10.2	0.0	2.6	1.3	1.3	3.2	0.0

tendency for nonspecific or pseudo-inhibition leading to considerable over-reporting of the presence of antibody (i.e. immunity). Neither of these laboratory errors would be picked up by the controls routinely performed with the test. It has been suggested that a known low-titered positive serum (titer 1:10–1:20) be included in each test as a positive control for the sensitivity of the test. False-positive reactions are much more complex and require thorough evaluation of the technique, especially the method of serum treatment employed.

An analysis of the intralaboratory agreement of the duplicate specimens in each laboratory gives additional evidence for concern. Table 7-III summarizes the agreement of duplicate specimens for each laboratory. Those duplicate specimens which differ in titer by two or more dilutions represent an estimate of probability for false-positive interpretations of paired serum antibody tests. These laboratories demonstrated reproducability ranging from 52 to 100 percent. Such information shakes one's confidence in the reliability of fourfold titer changes as being diagnostically significant. Recognizing that such "inherent" inaccuracies are seen even in laboratories highly experienced with rubella HI testing, we must look with great caution at results from other smaller and less experienced laboratories.

What can be done to minimize these "inherent" errors? The first step must be to recognize the factors which might contribute to such variation in results. Such factors include the method for serum treatment, uniformity of test procedure and reagents, quality of equipment used, and technician errors. Some investigators blame "inexperienced hands" as the major cause of test

TABLE 7-III

COLLABORATIVE RUBELLA HI STANDARDIZATION STUDY
ANALYSIS OF INTRALABORATORY TEST REPRODUCIBILITY

Agreement on Duplicate Spec*	Lab I		Lab II		Lab III Method A		Lab III Method B		Lab IV		Lab V Test 1		Lab V Test 2		Lab VI	
	No.	%	No.	%	No.	%	No.	%	No.	%	No.	%	No.	%	No.	%
Same titer	19	50.0	12	31.6	21	48.8	21	52.5	18	43.9	12	15.2	30	37.9	17	42.5
1 dilution apart	16	42.1	19	50.0	20	46.5	19	47.5	19	46.3	29	36.7	32	40.5	18	45.0
2 dilutions apart	3	7.9	6	15.8	2	4.7			2	4.9	13	16.5	2	4.9	5	12.5
3 dilutions apart			1	2.6					2	4.9	17	21.5	4	5.1		
4 dilutions apart											8	10.1				
Total no. of duplicates	38	100.0	38	100.0	43	100.0	40	100.0	41	100.0	79‡	100.0	79‡	100.0	40	100.0
Reproducibility†	92.1%		81.6%		95.3%		100.0%		90.2%		51.9%		78.4%		87.5%	

* Negative sera not included in analysis.
† Reproducibility defined as the percentage of duplicate specimens with titers differing by less than 2 twofold dilutions.
‡ Totals represent combined results of duplicate runs in each test.

inaccuracies. Although this undoubtedly is a major factor in some instances, the failures in reproducibility outlined in the above collaborative study could not be attributed to limitations in technical skill. Emphasis therefore has been directed toward evaluating all aspects of the procedure itself to detect and eliminate those factors which have contributed most heavily to the variability, and thus the reliability, of the HI test. The CDC rubella laboratory together with several other competent research laboratories are currently compiling comparative data on different diluent systems, various serum treatment methods, and erythrocyte types in an attempt to find the optimum methodology. Although no final conclusions can be made at this time on these studies, some of the preliminary observations will be summarized for this conference by the Ad Hoc Committee for Standardization of Rubella Techniques.

Another essential step toward developing technical competence in rubella laboratory testing is through an active program of laboratory training. This past Spring the CDC held a series of one-week training courses for personnel from state and city health departments. The Center also plans to conduct field courses in various parts of the country in an effort to upgrade the level of technical competence for rubella testing all over the country. It is hoped that this training on a national level will generate active training programs on the state and local levels and thus expand the laboratory capability for rubella testing.

Such training, whether it be on a national or local level, should be closely tied in with a program of proficiency testing. Periodic distribution of "unknowns" to participating laboratories allows one to monitor the general quality of rubella test performance by a laboratory, and problem areas can be more easily identified and appropriate corrective action taken. An active proficiency testing program has been a prominent feature of the CDC's relationship with the state health department laboratories.

The third general area of involvement of the public health service in improving the quality and reliability of rubella testing is in the area of reagent development and control. Commercial antigens and reagents for rubella HI or CF tests are now available from four companies in this country. The CDC has recently begun a voluntary quality testing program of premarketed rubella reagents with all four of these firms to insure that only satisfactory quality reagents be released for sale. Such cooperative efforts will help diminish inaccuracies resulting from impotent or poor quality reagents.

Information on the results of the quality control testing of premarketed rubella reagents will be disseminated periodically to all state public health laboratory directors by the CDC. In addition, the commercial companies will be permitted to package satisfactory reagents with an enclosed statement that they meet PHS recommended specifications.

Emphasis has been placed up to this point on rubella HI antibody testing. Little mention has been made in this discussion about other rubella laboratory techniques such as complement fixation, fluorescent antibody, or viral isolation methods.

Few diagnostic laboratories are adequately equipped or have reagents available for extending rubella testing beyond the HI test. Since in certain special situations these supplemental tests may be required for accurate and complete laboratory interpretation, it is essential that competent reference laboratory services be available to provide these more difficult laboratory "tools." The CDC Virus Reference Laboratory currently serves as the back-up for the State Public Health Laboratories. As better quality CF antigen becomes available at a reasonable cost, more laboratories, especially state laboratories, will be strongly encouraged to develop these services. But until such time when these reagents and tests are more widely available, efforts towards control and standardization of rubella laboratory testing will be focused almost entirely on the rubella HI test.

In conclusion, we have attempted to present some of the current views and problems concerning rubella laboratory testing as we see them from the federal level. It is clear that deficiencies in the rubella HI test currently exist in many laboratories. The U.S. Public Health Service has begun studies toward standardizing the rubella HI test procedure, has established a voluntary reagent quality control program with the commercial companies producing rubella reagents, and has provided technical training for many state and local health department laboratory personnel.

It is hoped that through developing guidelines and standards for rubella laboratory performance and insuring the availability of quality reagents we may move toward that goal of insuring accurate rubella diagnostic test be available to all.

REFERENCES

1. Halonen, P. E., Ryan, J. M., and Stewart, J. A.: Rubella hemagglutinin prepared with alkaline extraction of virus grown in suspension culture of BHK-21 cells. *Proc. Soc. Exp. Biol. Med.*, 125:162-167, 1967.
2. Stewart, G. L., Parkman, P. D., Hopps, H. E., Douglas, R. D., Hamilton, J. P., and Meyer, H. M., Jr.: Rubella-virus hemagglutination-inhibition test. *NEJM*, 276:554-557, 1967.
3. Cooper, L. Z., Matters, B., Rosenblum, J. K., and Krugman, S.: Experience with a modified rubella hemagglutination-inhibition antibody test. *JAMA*, 207:89-93, 1969.
4. Phillips, C. A., and O'Brien, L.: Evaluation of a macro-hemagglutination-inhibition kit for determining rubella antibody. *Am. J. Clin. Path.*, 51:295-297, 1969.
5. Peetermans, J., and Huygelen, C.: L'emploi d'hermaties de pigeons dans le test d'inhibition de l'hemagglutination de le rubeole. *Presse Med.*, 75:2177-2178, 1967.
6. Auletta, A. E., Gitnick, G. L., Whitmire, C. E., and Sever, J. L.: An improved diluent for rubella hemagglutination and hemagglutination-inhibition tests. *Appl. Microbiol.*, 16:691-694, 1968.

Chapter 8

THE INTERPRETATION OF LABORATORY DATA FOR THE DIAGNOSIS OF RUBELLA

STANLEY A. PLOTKIN

THE laboratory should be able to give the clinician assistance in interpretation of reports concerning serologic tests for rubella. It is quite obvious that physicians are frequently unable to understand laboratory reports without such assistance and equally obvious that the laboratory cannot interpret its own data without knowledge of the clinical circumstances. Therefore, a complete history of the patient and the circumstances must be made available to the laboratory at the time of submission of the first specimens for diagnosis of rubella, so that appropriate additional specimens can be requested, if needed.

Basically, there are four situations in which the laboratory might be asked for aid: (1) exposure of a pregnant woman to alleged rubella; (2) the presence of a rubella-like disease in any patient, particularly one who is also pregnant; (3) the past history of a recent rubella-like disease in a pregnant woman; (4) the presence of possible signs of rubella syndrome in an infant.

EXPOSURE OF A PREGNANT WOMAN TO ALLEGED RUBELLA

When a pregnant woman may have been exposed to rubella, a blood specimen should be obtained as soon as possible. It appears from studies of volunteers infected with wild virus, and also from investigations of attenuated vaccines, that antibodies are not elicited until about 14 days postinfection at the earliest. Ten days from the time of exposure appears to be a reasonably safe period during which a serum specimen will not yet contain antibodies stimulated by the exposure.

The hemagglutination-inhibition (HI) test will usually be used to test for immunity. If a woman has HI antibodies at the

76

time of exposure, one can interpret this fact either simplistically or sophisticatedly—not that the sophisticated way is necessarily preferable. In the simplistic view the possession of antibodies at titers even as low as ⅛ or ¼₀ means that a woman will not get clinical rubella. This rule has appeared to be valid in studies of volunteers inoculated with wild virus.

The sophisticate, however, will also ask what is the possibility of reinfection of immune individuals, particularly when titers are low; and if reinfection takes place, what is the risk to the fetus? Unfortunately, complete answers are not available to these questions. It appears from the studies of Schiff, Portnoy, Horstmann, and many other laboratories that reinfection does take place with some frequency. Isolated cases of second clinical attacks of rubella have even been recorded (Public Health Working Party). Reinfection (as determined by presence of virus in the nasopharynx) may also take place in the absence of an increase in antibodies. Whether reinfection of the mother poses a hazard to the fetus is conjectural. All that can be said is that no evidence has been produced proving that it is dangerous. In the present state of our knowledge therefore, women with moderate or high antibody titers at the time of exposure can be reassured. Those with low titers had better be retested a month later. In our laboratory, we have decided that 1:10 or 1:20 are low titers, and women with these titers are retested.

If a pregnant woman is seronegative at the time of exposure she must of course be considered at risk of infection and a second specimen must certainly be obtained. The minimum period for the collection of a second specimen is 21 days, although blood collected as early as 14 days postexposure may have antibody and waiting for 28 days would perhaps be safer in order to detect late rises. A number of studies of natural rubella have shown that HI antibody has always appeared by 28 days postinfection.

When the second specimen still is negative for antibodies, we can conclude that the woman has not been infected. Implicit in this conclusion is that belief that natural rubella infection always elicits an immune response which reaches levels of at least ⅛ in the HI. So far no exception to this rule has been recorded.

If the second specimen shows seroconversion, and the woman

TABLE 8-I

EXPOSURE TO RUBELLA

Serum Specimens		Interpretation
1	2 (28 d*)	
Pos.	Pos.→	Immune to rubella
Pos.	Pos.↑	Reinfection rubella?
Neg.	Neg.	No rubella
Neg.	Pos.	Rubella

* Post-exposure.
Pos. = rubella antibodies present.
Neg. = no rubella antibodies present.

has had clinical rubella in the interval, few would argue against the advisability of abortion. Estimates of the risk of abnormality differ quantitatively, but the British, Swedish, and NIH collaborative studies all show a marked risk of abnormality during the first 12 weeks of pregnancy. There is also general agreement that the fetus is still in some danger through the sixteenth week. Sever, Dudgeon, and their respective collaborators have also observed congenitally defective infants who were the result of maternal rubella later in the second trimester.

Whether subclinical rubella presents as much risk to the fetus as does clinical rubella is a matter of some dispute. It is not possible to give a quantitative answer to this question, but there is no doubt that many cases of congenital rubella syndrome have followed inapparent rubella. Therefore, advice in favor of abortion is justified.

Table 8-I summarizes the approach to a patient exposed to rubella.

Before leaving this category, the influence of gamma globulin must be mentioned. If a large amount of gamma globulin was administered to the patient after exposure, caution should be used in interpreting the results of testing the second specimen, since low titers of passive antibody may be present for several weeks after inoculation. The British Public Health Laboratory Working Party on Rubella showed the presence of HI titers as high as ¹⁄₆₄ two to three weeks postinoculation of 750 mg of gamma globulin.

RUBELLA-LIKE DISEASE

The patient who develops signs of rubella should of course be seen by a physician as soon as possible. Swabs for virus isolation and a first blood specimen should be obtained at that time. Experience during the 1964 epidemic showed that nasal swabs, even from the turbinates alone, are more likely to be positive than pharyngeal swabs. Therefore, both nose and throat swabs should be taken.

The acute blood specimen may also be used to test for viremia, but the incidence of recovery is so small once the rash has appeared that attempts to isolate virus from serum are not worthwhile. It may be, based on recent evidence, that washed white cells would be a more fruitful source of rubella virus in blood.

If inoculated into the standard tissue culture systems, specimens for virus isolation may not give positive results for several weeks. Newer and faster methods have been developed. For example, Haire has successfully stained smears obtained by nasopharyngeal swabs with fluorescent antibody against rubella. Hemadsorption-inhibition tests have also been applied to rapid identification. Virus growing in tissue culture cells can be stained by fluorescence or their ability to produce specific hemadsorption or hemagglutinin can be tested.

The isolation of a rubella virus from the pregnant patient will be regarded by most observers as sufficient reason for an abortion. In contrast, negative culture, particularly if taken more than 24 hours after the onset of the rash, when virus becomes more difficult to isolate, cannot be considered as certain evidence against abortion.

If the patient has no HI antibodies at the time of the rash, the second specimen becomes crucial. It may be taken as early as a week after the onset of rash, and if then positive, rubella has certainly occurred. If negative, a third specimen should be obtained after another week. In other words, most patients will have seroconverted by one week after illness, but some will take two weeks.

Serial negative tests, that is, titers less than ⅛ at two or more

TABLE 8-II

RASH DISEASE IN PREGNANCY

Serum Specimens		Interpretation
1	2 (7-14 d*)	
Neg.	Neg.	No rubella
Neg.	Pos.	Rubella
Pos.	Pos. ↑	Rubella
Pos.	Pos.→	Other tests must be done to detect recent infection

* After onset of rash.

weeks after the rash, are incontrovertible evidence that rubella has not in fact occurred, but has been mimicked by some other infection.

Often antibodies will be already present at the time of the rash. If that is the case, a second blood specimen two weeks later is necessary in order to search for a diagnostic titer rise. Tests other than the HI, in particular CF and immunofluorescence, may be useful, since they are frequently negative days after the HI has become positive, which makes the demonstration of a seroconversion easier.

In addition, techniques designed to measure the amount of newly synthesized macroglobulin rubella antibody are helpful. Destruction of macroglobulins by 2-mercaptoethanol or density gradient centrifugation of serum are the techniques most used. If 50 percent or more of antibody can be shown to be in the macroglobulin fraction, then recent infection is probable.

Of course, in some cases in which antibody is present at the time of rash, reinfection rather than primary infection may be taking place. In this connection, it must be remembered that secondary immune responses bring forth IgG antibodies. Therefore, fractionation of antibodies may help distinguish a primary from a secondary response. Table 8-II summarizes the approach to the situation of a pregnant woman with a rash.

HISTORY OF RECENT RUBELLA

This is the most difficult and surely the most annoying of all categories. The typical case is of the woman who did not know she was pregnant at the time of an illness with rash and who consults her physician weeks after the attack of possible rubella. Virus isolation is hopeless in these cases. If the rash has occurred within two weeks of the first blood specimen there is a good possibility of showing a fourfold increase in the HI titer. After two weeks, such a demonstration becomes much harder. Therefore, it is in this situation that the use of CF, immunofluorescence, and macroglobulin antibody tests are most helpful. In relation to CF testing, it should be noted that the alkaline extracted CF antigen is more sensitive than the cell pack antigen, but because of this fact the latter has the advantage of showing late rises more clearly.

In relation to diagnostic problems in all of the three categories mentioned, I would like to stress the value of testing specimens from the alleged source of rubella. For example, a woman was sent to us recently whose one-year-old child had a rash-disease diagnosed as rubella, subsequent to which she discovered that she was pregnant. Two serial HI tests showed rubella antibodies in her serum at a level of $\frac{1}{80}$. An abortion was considered because her physician thought it was too late to be sure that she had been immune at the time of exposure. However, a specimen taken from the infant failed to reveal antibodies, proving that the woman had not in fact been exposed to rubella. We have frequently found that such additional epidemiologic data assist in preventing needless concern. The supposed index case is often an infant or preschool child, perhaps the woman's own, and determination of their serological status is indicated. Table 8-III summarizes the approach to diagnosis of rubella in the past.

TABLE 8-III

HISTORY OF RASH IN PREGNANCY

Serum Specimens		
1	2	Interpretation
Neg.	Neg.	No rubella
Neg.	Pos.	Rubella
Pos.	Pos. ↑	Rubella
Pos.	Pos.→	Other tests must be done*

* CF and FA tests, search for IgM rubella antibodies, test of serum from source of alleged rubella.

CONGENITAL RUBELLA

The confirmation of a clinical diagnosis of intrauterine rubella infection must be analyzed by separation of the patients into three age groups: those less than 6 months, 6 months to 5 years, and more than 5 years.

The infant less than 6 months old, normal or otherwise, will probably have maternal antibodies to rubella. To distinguish normal passive antibody from active, three procedures may be followed: (1) The infant's and the mother's blood can be titrated simultaneously. If the infant's titer does not progressively drop below the maternal titer as he gets older, active infection is probable. The half-life of maternally derived rubella antibodies in the infant is about one month. (2) IgM rubella antibody can be searched for in the infant's serum, which if present, can only be the product of the infant's own lymphoid cells. (3) Nasopharyngeal swabs should be taken for virus isolation. The recovery of rubella virus, particularly if repeated, would be conclusive proof of congenital infection.

Because the rate of recovery of rubella virus from the nasopharynx falls rapidly with increasing age, the diagnosis of intrauterine rubella after six months is primarily serologic. To be sure, virus should be sought for in the nasopharynx, but positive results will be sparse. More useful is the culture of cerebrospinal fluid, which may remain positive for long periods. Even more helpful is the culture of cataractous lens, which may contain virus long after it has disappeared from other sites.

Nevertheless, the demonstration of rubella antibodies in the infant's serum beyond the time that they can be accounted for by passive transfer and in the absence of postnatal exposure, is the cornerstone of the diagnosis of congenital rubella until the child enters school. In our series and those of others, 95 percent of children with rubella syndrome have had HI antibodies. That means, of course, that conversely, 5 percent are negative, so that some reservation has to be made about excluding the diagnosis of rubella syndrome if antibodies are absent. The use of additional serologic tests is not particularly helpful since the CF re-

TABLE 8-IV

DIAGNOSIS OF CONGENITAL RUBELLA

Less than 6 months of age:
  NP swabs pos.
  IgM rubella antibodies
  Compare maternal and infant titer

6 months to school age:
  Virus may be in lens or in CSF
  Pos. HI antibody

sponse in congenital disease is variable and the other tests parallel the HI.

When children reach school, where postnatal exposure to rubella is frequent, the serologic diagnosis of rubella syndrome becomes impossible. In this regard, it is interesting that long-term follow-up data from Australia suggests that an increasing percentage of rubella syndrome patients become seronegative as they grow older. Table 8-IV summarizes the tools for verification of congenital rubella.

Chapter 9

SEROLOGIC RESPONSES AFTER PRIMARY INFECTION AND AFTER REINFECTION WITH RUBELLA VIRUS

Dorothy M. Horstmann

THE patterns of response in terms of the four antibodies commonly tested for, hemagglutination-inhibition (HI), complement fixing (CF), and neutralizing antibodies, as well as those detected by fluorescence techniques (FA), are summarized in Figure 9-1. These antibodies have been reviewed by previous participants in this symposium to (1) the time of their appearance, (2) their sensitivity in detecting infection, and (3) their relative usefulness in diagnostic problems and in serologic surveys to de-

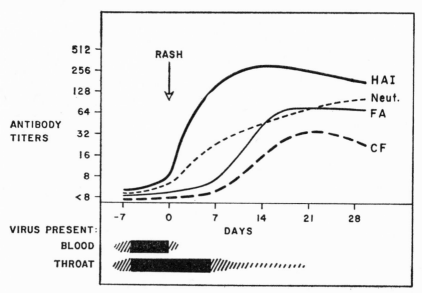

Figure 9-1. Antibody responses to primary infection with rubella virus. HI, hemagglutination-inhibition; Neut., neutralizing; FA, fluorescent and CF, complement fixing antibodies.

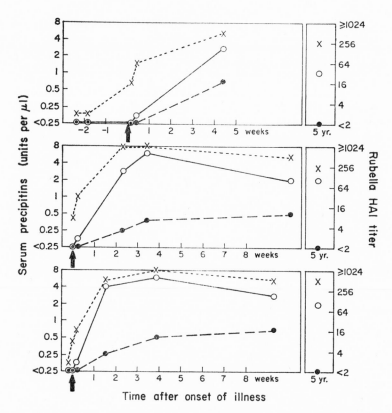

Figure 9-2. Serum antibody responses over a 5-year period in 3 children with rubella. Arrows indicate time of appearance of rash. HI antibody (x); anti-theta precipitin (O); anti-iota precipitin (●). From Le Bouvier, G. (2).

termine the immune status of population groups. I have nothing to add on these points and will not repeat what has already been said.

There are, however, additional serologic responses to rubella virus, including anti-precipitin, anti-platelet aggregation, and hemadsorption inhibiting antibodies. Small-size, nonviral, soluble antigens which can be detected in the medium from rubella-infected cell cultures by immuno-diffusion have been described by Schmidt and Styk (1), LeBouvier (2), and by Halonen *et al* (3).

Dr. LeBouvier, working in our laboratory,* has shown that following infection antibodies to two of these antigens (which he has designated theta and iota) appear regularly in the serum. Figure 9-2 shows the time of their appearance in three representative patients in relation to onset of rash. The persistence of these antibodies over a five-year period is also shown, and HI responses are included for comparison. Both types of antiprecipitin antibodies were demonstrated in the sera of all three patients: anti-theta appeared earlier, soon after HI antibodies were detectable; it rose more rapidly and to a higher titer than anti-iota which was delayed about seven days. Five years later, anti-theta and HI titers of these same patients were maintained at relatively high levels, but anti-iota antibodies had completely disappeared. The presence of substantial amounts of anti-theta with little or no anti-iota, with no change in either antibody over a few days, would therefore indicate previous rubella infection and immunity (2).

Another soluble rubella antigen, platelet aggregation or PA, has been described by Vaheri *et al* (4). Following infection, antibodies against this antigen appear in the serum at about the same time as CF antibodies, but they rise to higher titers. The levels are particularly high in patients who have post-rubella thrombocytopenia. According to Vaheri *et al*, PA antigen-antibody complexes are capable of aggregating human platelets, which may be part of the explanation of the pathogenesis of this complication (4).

Another characteristic of rubella virus, namely its ability to hemadsorb a variety of erythrocytes (5), forms the basis of the hemadsorption-inhibition test which has been described by Lennette and Schmidt (6). This appears to be a sensitive system for antibody detection, comparable to the HI test, but having no particular advantage over the HI method for serologic work. The main use of the hemadsorption technique may be in the isolation of rubella virus which can then be identified rapidly by means of the hemadsorption inhibition test (5).

The discussion of serologic responses elsewhere in this sym-

* Personal work supported by rubella contract #PH-43-68-1037.

posium has focussed primarily on natural infection in completely susceptible individuals without previous experience with rubella. I should like to turn now to a consideration of serologic reactions of partially immune persons who experience reinfection when exposed naturally or artificially to wild rubella virus.

Our first exploration of this subject was an experimental one, using chimpanzees (7). These animals proved quite susceptible and on primary infection had viremia and shed virus from the throat for some days. None of the five tested developed any clinical evidence of rubella. All responded with neutralizing CF, and

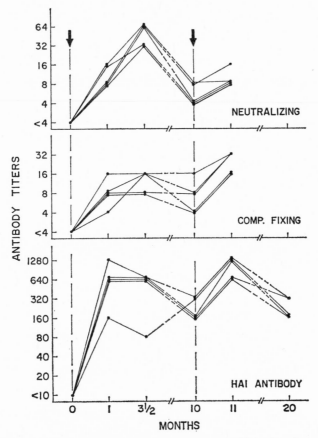

Figure 9-3. Antibody responses of 5 chimpanzees following first infection with rubella virus and virus challenge 10 months later. Arrows indicate time of virus administration. From Horstmann, D., *et al* (7).

HI antibodies (Fig. 9-3). Ten months after their first infection, they were challenged with either homologous or heterologous wild virus (intramuscularly and by throat swab) and all exhibited antibody boosts. However, no virus was detected in the blood or in throat swabs of any of the animals. We interpreted these results as indicating that reinfection had occurred, but virus multiplication was at such a low level that we could not detect it by currently available techniques.

Reinfection in persons who have previously had natural rubella has also been documented in several studies. We observed two individuals with naturally acquired antibody who on exposure in an epidemic in a closed population exhibited fourfold or greater rises in HI and neutralizing antibody titers. Others have reported similar observations. The overall available evidence suggests that this happens rarely, however, and in general the presence of even low level antibody acquired by natural infection seems to protect against reinfection.

Turning to the problem of reinfection in *vaccinees*, here there are data based on artificial challenge and from observations on the resistance of vaccinated persons exposed to naturally occurring rubella. A word about the serologic responses to attenuated rubella virus vaccines is necessary to interpret these data. As Dr. Lennette stated (Ch. 3), there are differences between the antibody patterns following naturally occurring rubella and vaccine-induced infection. First, HI titers are considerably higher in the natural infection, four- to eight-fold in general. Secondly, although CF and FA antibodies appear regularly after natural infection, after vaccination they are either absent, or present at quite low levels, depending on the nature and sensitivity of the antigen used in the test (6, 8). It is not yet clear whether these differences in immune response are entirely quantitative or whether they are to some extent qualitative as well. In any event, using selected antigens the CF and FA tests can be useful in following vaccinees to determine reinfection rates in those exposed to natural rubella.

The responses of vaccinees challenged by intranasal instillation of low passage wild virus have been examined by several groups of investigators. Meyer and Parkman (9) first demonstrated significant HI antibody rises in two of five vaccinees challenged with wild virus. In studies reported by Wilkins *et al* (10) four of eight HPV77 vaccine immunes responded with inapparent infections resulting in marked rises in HI titer and the appearance of CF antibodies. These investigators also demonstrated that on exposure to natural rubella, seven of eight vaccinees in a closed population were reinfected as evidenced by significant HI antibody rises, and the development of CF antibody. Similar observations have been made by Schiff *et al* (11). In all of these studies virus shedding from the throat has been demonstrated in some of the reinfected individuals, but none had detectable viremia, and none had any clinical signs of rubella.

We recently undertook field studies on vaccinees exposed to wild rubella virus under natural conditions (12). The subjects were military recruits of the All-Hawaiian Company who had been bled and vaccinated with the Cendehill strain some two to three months before the company was formed at Fort Ord, California. This phase of the study was carried out by our colleague Dr. Scott Halstead, of the University of Hawaii. Hawaiian recruits were chosen because of the documented high susceptibility rates among young adult residents of the Hawaiian Islands (13, 14) and the regular occurrence of rubella each year in the All-Hawaiian Company at Fort Ord. As it turned out, fifteen of the vaccinees proved susceptible at the time of vaccination, and all seroconverted. Their postvaccinal HI titers ranged from 1:16 to 1:128, with a geometric mean titer (GMT) of 34.2. Six of the 15 developed CF antibodies as a result of vaccination (15), with titers of 1:8 or 1:16.

Approximately three weeks after arrival at Fort Ord clinical rubella appeared in the All-Hawaiian Company (Table 9-I). At the time the company consisted of 190 men. Of these, 26 were

TABLE 9-I

RUBELLA EPIDEMIC AMONG 190 RECRUITS OF THE ALL-HAWAIIAN
COMPANY, FORT ORD, CALIFORNIA

	Number	% of Total Company	Infected Number	%
Susceptible	26	13.6	26	100
Vaccine immunes	15	7.9	12	80
Natural immunes	149	78.4	2	1.3

susceptible, antibody negatives; 15 were vaccinees and antibody positive; and 149 were natural immunes. In spite of the 86% immunity rate when the virus was introduced, it spread rapidly through the company and all 26 susceptibles became infected: 17 had inapparent infections and nine developed clinical rubella with rash, a ratio of inapparent to apparent infection of 1.9:1. The 15 vaccinees and 149 natural immunes thus had a significant exposure. Their reinfection rates are shown in Table 9-I. Twelve of the vaccinees or 80 percent had inapparent infections. The HI antibody GMT of these men before exposure was 33.4, while afterwards it was 236 (Table 9-II). Two of the 149 natural immunes also showed HI antibody rises, in both cases from levels of 1:16 to 1:16 to 1:128. Virus isolation studies on the two groups are currently under way, but results are not yet available.

As to the CF antibody responses, all but one of the vaccinees who were reinfected (as indicated by increases in HI titer) also had fourfold CF rises or developed CF antibody. An additional two men who had only twofold rises in HI nevertheless had sharp CF responses, indicating that they also were reinfected.

Figure 9-4 shows diagrammatically the serologic responses of two men, one who experienced a primary infection and had clinical rubella with rash, and the other, a vaccinee who became reinfected. The patterns are similar. The clinical disease was accompanied by seroconversion as measured by both HI and CF antibody responses, the peak HI titer being 1:256, and the CF, 1:128. Characteristically, the appearance of CF antibody lagged behind that of NAI antibody.

TABLE 9-II

HEMAGGLUTINATION-INHIBITION (HI) ANTIBODY RESPONSES OF
RECRUITS EXPOSED DURING A RUBELLA EPIDEMIC

| | No. | Geometric Mean Titers | |
		Before Exposure	After Exposure
Susceptible	26	0	197
Vaccinees	15		
Reinfected	12	33.4	236
Not reinfected	3	39	48
Natural immunes	149		
Reinfected	2	16	128
Not reinfected	147	97.5	97.5

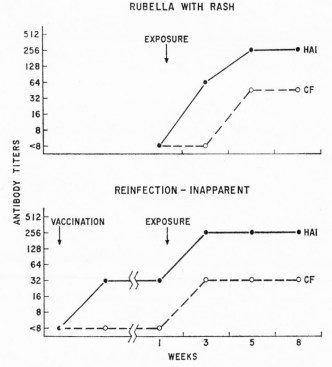

Figure 9-4. Antibody responses of two recruits infected with rubella virus.

In the lower panel of Figure 9-4 representative results with one of the vaccinees is shown. At the time of exposure to wild rubella virus this man had an HI titer of 1:32 and no detectable CF antibody. As a result of reinfection, his HI titer rose to 1:256, and he developed CF antibody to a level of 1:32. We have not yet tested for FA and antiprecipitin antibodies, but based on previous experience one would expect rises in these, too.

From this and other studies, then, it appears that the serologic responses following natural *reinfection* are similar in quantity and quality to those associated with primary experience with wild rubella virus. The striking antibody increases in the vaccinees whom we studied suggests that they experienced more than simple slight multiplication of virus in the pharynx. What the data on reinfection mean in relation to efforts to control rubella by immunization of the childhood population is not an easy question to answer. They do suggest that herd immunity is not going to be easily achieved, and they raise some doubts as to how sturdy the immunity of a young adult vaccinated in childhood will be as compared to the resistance of one who experienced natural infection in the past. This point is highly pertinent since rubella is unique in that our main concern is not the vaccinee, but the fetus to whom the infection may be transmitted at some future date, perhaps many years hence. Even if one is optimistic as to the eventual outcome of widespread immunization, continued surveillance of the serologic status of vaccinated populations, using HI, CF, and FA antibody methods would seem to be indicated for some time to come. By such means it should be possible to follow the circulation of wild virus and to assess the impact of immunization on this important aspect of the rubella problem.

REFERENCES

1. Schmidt, N. J., and Styk, B.: Immunodiffusion reactions with rubella antigens. *J. Immunol.*, 101:210-216, 1968.
2. Le Bouvier, G. L.: Precipitinogens of rubella-virus-infected cells. *Proc. Soc. Exp. Biol. Med.*, 130:51-54, 1969.
3. Halonen, P.: In Discussion, International Conference on Rubella Immunization. *Am. J. Dis. Child.*, 118:146, 1969.
4. Vaheri, A., Vesikari, T., Penttinen, K., and Myllylä, G.: Soluble rubella antigens, platelet aggregation, and post-rubella thrombocytopenia. In *International Symposium on Rubella Vaccines*, Symp. Series Immunobiol. Stand., Vol. 11, pp. 107-108. Basel/New York, S. Karger, 1969.
5. Perlino, C. A., and Isacson, P.: Direct hemadsorption by cell cultures infected with rubella virus. *Am. J. Dis. Child.*, 118:83-88, 1969.
6. Lennette, E., and Schmidt, N. J.: Complement fixing and fluorescent antibody responses to an attenuated rubella virus vaccine. To be published.
7. Horstmann, D. M., Pajot, T. G., and Liebhaber, H.: Epidemiology of rubella. Subclinical infection and occurrence of reinfection. *Am. J. Dis. Child.*, 118:133-136, 1969.
8. Monto, A. S., Cavallaro, J. J., and Brown, G. C.: Attenuated rubella vaccination in families: observations on the lack of fluorescent antibody response, and on the use of blood collected on filter paper discs in the hemagglutination-inhibition test. *J. Lab. Clin. Med.*, 74:98-102, 1969.

9. Meyer, H. M., Jr., *et al:* Clinical studies with experimental live rubella virus vaccine (Strain HPV77). Evaluation of vaccine-induced immunity. *Am. J. Dis. Child.,* 115:648-654, 1968.

10. Wilkins, J., Leedom, J. M., Portnoy, B., and Salvatore, M. A.: Reinfection with rubella virus despite live vaccine induced immunity. *Am. J. Dis. Child.,* 118:275-294, 1969.

11. Schiff, G., Donath, R., and Rotte, T.: Experimental rubella studies. I. Clinical and laboratory features of infection caused by the Brown strain of rubella virus. II. Artificial challenge studies of adult rubella vaccinees. *Am. J. Dis. Child.,* 118:269-274, 1969.

12. Horstmann, D. M., Liebhaber, H., Rosenberg, D., and Halstead, S.: Unpublished observations.

13. Sever, J. L., *et al:* Rubella antibody among pregnant women in Hawaii. *Am. J. Obstet. Gynec.,* 92:1006-1009, 1965.

14. Halstead, S. B., and Diwan, A. R.: Rubella susceptibility among adults in Hawaii. Differences by sex and ethnic group. *Hawaiian Med. J.* In press.

15. Liebhaber, H., Riordan, J. T., and Horstmann, D. M.: Replication of rubella virus in a continuous line of African green monkey kidney cells (Vero). *Proc. Soc. Exp. Biol. & Med.,* 125:636-643, 1967.

Chapter 10

IMMUNOLOGY OF RUBELLA

CHARLES A. ALFORD, JR.

R UBELLA infections acquired in the postnatal period produce acute diseases which are clinically variable and are limited by the host defense mechanisms to a two- to three-week interval, at least, as defined by viral excretion. In contrast when the conceptus is invaded in the early stages of pregnancy the infection may become a chronic process. Virus persists in the placenta and fetus throughout the remaining months of intrauterine life and, in a majority of afflicted infants, viral excretion can be demonstrated for a number of months following delivery. Though persistence may be prolonged in areas such as the eye and brain, presumably because they are protected from the full force of the developing immunologic mechanisms, viral excretion is generally brought under control within the first year after delivery of infants with the classic rubella syndrome. Attempts to explain these differences in the pattern of viral infection with congenitally and postnatally acquired rubella have focused attention on the maturation of host defense mechanisms *in utero* and during early infancy. At present, no single missing factor has been found to explain the chronicity of the fetal infection, but considerable information has been acquired about the immunology of naturally occurring rubella infections. This will be briefly reviewed here as outlined in Table 10-I.

As with most acute viral infections, both humoral and cellular factors and their interrelation are considered to be important in resisting and overcoming the infection. These include, under the former heading, primarily antibody production, its qualitative and quantitative nature and its relation to the introduction of virus. Perhaps of more importance in clearing the acute infection, once it has become established, are the cellular immune factors including interferon, activated small lymphocytes and in-

94

TABLE 10-I

IMMUNOLOGY OF NATURALLY OCCURRING FETAL INFECTIONS

A. Humoral Factors
   Transfer maternal antibody
   Production of fetal antibody

B. Cellular factors
   Production of fetal interferon
   Role of small lymphocyte
   Role of innate cellular factors

nate biochemical cellular factors. With rubella infections acquired in the earliest stages of pregnancy, one is concerned with the activation of each of these components in the infected mother, the role of the placenta in transferring humoral factors from mother to fetus and, finally, with the development and efficacy of each of the immunologic components in the maturing fetus. In this respect, more information has been gained in recent years on humoral factors. Therefore, these will be considered initially in greater detail as shown in Table 10-II.

First, rubella antibody levels were determined in sera collected from young fetuses, infants and children with or without congenital rubella infections. Antibody is detectable in fetal sera from both infected and control material as early as the eleventh week of gestation, and also is present at birth in both of these populations. After delivery, levels of maternally transferred antibody decline and disappear in the first six months in the control population while persistently elevated titers are detected for

TABLE 10-II

RUBELLA NEUTRALIZING ANTIBODY STUDIES

| | Age Distribution | | | |
Patients	11-16 Week Fetus	1 Day-6 Mos.	6-12 Mos.	1-5 Yrs.
Congenital Rubella				
Neut. AB+	7	17	7	11
Neut. AB–	0	0	0	2
Controls				
Neut. AB+	8	36	0	1
Neut. AB–	0	6	10	18

years in sera from infants and children with the rubella syndrome.
Such data clearly indicate that immunologic tolerance, in the
classic sense, cannot explain the chronicity of fetal infection following maternal rubella. Instead, even though the fetus has been
invaded in the earliest stages of embryogenesis, the virus is recognized as a foreign antigen and antibody production begins either
in utero or postnatally.

Data from the uninfected control fetuses also indicate that maternal rubella antibody can be transferred across the normal placenta in the early stages of gestation. Because of the probability
that the rubella-infected placenta might also transfer maternal
antibody, these data do not permit a decision as to whether or not
fetal antibody production can be elicited by the infected conceptus. To gain insight into this problem, the quantitative relations and physicochemical properties of the antibody in these
and matched as well as other appropriate maternal sera were
compared and related to virologic events. The data in Figure 10-1

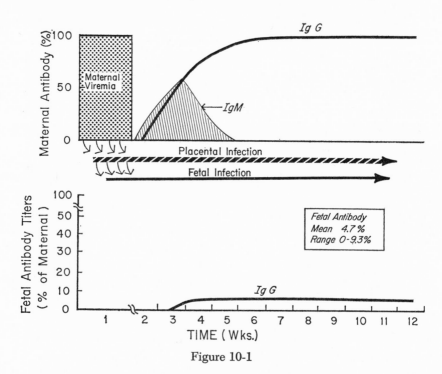

Figure 10-1

summarizes the virologic and immunologic findings encountered during the first 16 to 20 weeks of pregnancy following a typical case of maternal rubella. Virus appears in the blood of the mother approximately one week before the onset of rash. During this period, antibody cannot be demonstrated by standard serologic methods and, if present, is obviously unable to limit the spread of virus via the bloodstream. Shortly after the beginning of the rash, antibody appears in the serum of the mother and the viremia clears. Depending upon the type of serologic method used for demonstration, it reaches a peak within one week to one month after the disappearance of rash. During the first few weeks following initiation of the response, the maternal antibody pool is composed of IgG as well as a significant but unknown proportion of high molecular weight, 2 mercaptoethanol sensitive IgM moieties. It is of interest that detection of this latter variety of antibody has been employed to diagnose recently acquired rubella at a time when the results of total antibody determinations in the pregnant woman have proven inconclusive. After the first month, the persistent maternal antibody is predominantly, if not exclusively, IgG, a variety which, unlike IgM, can be transferred to the human fetus for protective purpose.

During the course of the viremia in the pregnant female, the placenta can become infected and remain so for prolonged periods in spite of the subsequent development of high levels of antibody in the maternal circulation. The infected placenta, which normally serves as a natural protective barrier for the human fetus, could then provide a seeding source of virus for the subsequent development of a chronic fetal infection. Though not yet conclusively established, epidemiologic and virologic data suggest that this sequence of events may be influenced by the age of the conceptus at the time of maternal rubella, even within the confines of the first 20 weeks of gestation.

At least two weeks, and perhaps even earlier, after the subsidence of the rash in the mother, low levels of rubella neutralizing antibody can be detected in sera collected from the infected fetuses and these appear to remain relatively unchanged even as long as 12 weeks following the disappearance of symptoms. Titers of rubella neutralizing antibody in fetal sera range from 2.5 to 9 and average only 4.5 percent of those in the maternal sera. In order to determine if rubella infection of the placenta would interfere with the transfer of maternal antibody, levels of polio antibody were evaluated in these same sera. It was present in approximately the same proportion as the rubella antibody. In addition, similarly low levels of both rubella and polio antibody were demonstrated in fetal sera from the control uninfected population.

In sera from both the control and rubella infected fetuses, quantities of total IgG were present which approximated 10 percent of those in the maternal sera and neither IgM nor IgA was demonstrated. According to immunoprecipitation and ultracentrifugal analysis, the antibodies present in all the fetal sera were IgG; there was no evidence of high molecular weight IgM antibody. From these studies it was concluded that the antibody present in fetal sera in the first 16 to 18 weeks following rubella infection of the conceptus is primarily of maternal origin.

Though IgM producing cells are present in human fetus as early as 10.5 weeks of gestation they apparently cannot produce sufficient quantities of specific antibody to maintain significant serum levels even in the face of stimulation by persistent rubella viral infection. The normal mechanisms necessary for the transfer of maternal antibody are likewise inefficient in this early stage of gestation. The net result is that weeks after peak levels have been reached in the mother, very low levels of antibody are maintained in serum of the infected fetus. By allowing the virus to gain a stronger foothold in the early stages of gestation, perhaps the inadequate fetal production and placental transfer mechanisms do, indeed, contribute to the chronicity of the fetal infection (Fig. 10-2).

Most likely due to the continuing normal maturational processes the capacity for fetal antibody production and placental transfer of maternal antibody becomes much more efficient as pregnancy advances beyond 18 to 20 weeks of gestation. For example, in the normal human fetus, serum IgG levels which reflect placental transfer mechanisms begin to increase markedly around 26 weeks gestation. Prior to this period, levels in the serum from normal fetuses approximate 10 to 20 percent of the

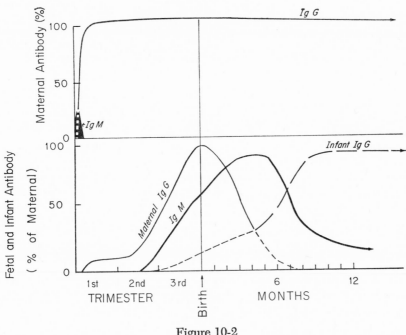

Figure 10-2

maternal values, but after 26 weeks gestation they rapidly increase to reach values comparable to those in the maternal serum.
We find that specific IgG rubella hemagglutination-inhibition
(HI) antibody follows this same pattern of intrauterine development in normal pregnancies. In pregnancies wherein the conceptus is infected by rubella virus in the first trimester (as noted
in Fig. 10-2), high levels of specific IgG, specific rubella and polio
antibodies which are comparable to those in the maternal serum
are detectable in umbilical cord sera collected from the chronically infected newborns. Since the placental transfer mechanisms
for IgG polio antibody remain intact in spite of chronic rubella
infection of the placenta, it is reasonable to assume that these
same mechanisms are capable of transferring the maternal IgG
rubella antibody later in gestation. If the quantitative parallelism
holds, then the major portion of IgG rubella antibody present
in the circulation of rubella infected newborns is likely of maternal origin. The fact that levels of IgG rubella antibody appear

to decline in the early months after delivery in a manner similar to that seen with the catabolism of maternally transferred antibody is further evidence for this suggestion.

However, some of the IgG rubella antibody present at birth may be contributed by infected fetus itself; IgG producing cells have been demonstrated in the tissue of normal human fetuses as early as 12 weeks of gestation and they apparently normally increase in number as gestation progresses. With herpetic infections of the human fetus, the number of these cells increases markedly and specific fetal IgG antibody has been demonstrated with other forms of antigenic stimulation. The possibility of fetal IgG antibody production with rubella infection has not yet been adequately examined.

Because specific IgM and IgA antibodies do not normally cross the placenta, they represent better markers than IgG for fetal antibody production. Though neither of these antibody types can be detected in sera in the early course of the fetal infection, significant levels of IgM rubella antibody can be detected at birth, even in very small prematurely born infected neonates. The accumulation of this material in the serum of the fetus occurs during a period when there is little or none of this antibody available in the maternal circulation for possible placental transfer. Thus, there appears to be an increasing capacity for fetal IgM antibody production as pregnancy progresses. In some cases, the antigenic stimulus provided by the infection is sufficient to cause premature manufacture of IgA *in utero* and elevated levels of this material can also be demonstrated at delivery.

In the first three to five months after delivery of a rubella-infected neonate, levels of IgM antibody can increase while IgG antibody diminishes. IgM can even become the dominant variety during this period. Later in the first year, presumably as the capacity for IgG production increases, the pattern is once again reversed. In spite of these constant changes in the molecular varieties that constitute the antibody pool in the first year following delivery of an infected infant, the level of total antibody which is equal to or in excess of that in the maternal serum remains virtually unchanged. In the majority of infants with the rubella syndrome, high levels of antibody are maintained for a number of years while in some they disappear at variable intervals beginning as early as 1.5 years after delivery. The reasons for the differences in antibody persistence are presently unknown but suggest varying degrees of substantial antigenic stimulation.

The stimulus provided by the chronic congenital infection is not only sufficient to provoke specific intrauterine antibody production but is also of such a magnitude in many cases that it causes sustained elevations in the total amount of three major circulating immunoglobulins. When the data for levels of IgM globulin in sera collected from congenitally infected neonates are compared to control values, IgM levels in infected infants, particularly those with congenital rubella, may be elevated at birth. If not, they increase at a more rapid rate in the neonatal period and are often sustained for many months postnatally. In fact, total IgM levels may remain markedly elevated even during the period when specific IgM antibody appears to be diminishing. At variable intervals during the course of infection, total IgG and IgA production apparently can be increased as well and elevated levels of these immunoglobulins may be maintained throughout early infancy and even longer. Such data as these suggest that a state of hypersensitivity as regards homologous antibody production exists in many patients as a result of the chronic congenital infection. In contrast in a few, the congenital infection may interfere with normal sequence of development of the immunologic process and result in a gammaglobulinemia or various types of dysgammaglobulinemia, including isolated IgA deficiencies. These states may alter the clinical cause in the postnatal period favoring an increased number of secondary bacterial infections. In addition, infected infants who are producing rubella antibody and increased amounts of immunoglobulin may show a reduced antibody responsiveness to the administration of heterologous antigens. Thus, when finally viewed *in toto*, the immunologic capacity of the classic type of rubella syndrome may be found to be deficient as regards the ability to produce antibody against other invading organisms.

Since viral excretion in congenital rubella may continue for many months after adequate amounts and types of specific antibody have been produced, obviously deficiencies in other immunologic factors must be sought to explain the chronicity of fetal infection. In recent years, the role of other cellular factors, particularly interferon and the small lymphocyte, have been examined in this regard.

It is generally thought that the embryo of most species is either incompetent or markedly deficient in its capacity to produce interferon in response to a viral infection, although this point has not been systematically studied in human fetuses because of the obvious technical difficulties encountered. In addition, rubella virus is known to be a relatively poor stimulator of interferon production, at least in most vitro cell systems, including human embryonic cells of many types. From this data, it is tempting to conclude that chronicity of the fetal infection in congenital rubella may be, in part, due to inadequate interferon production *in utero*. Investigators in Houston have been unable to demonstrate interferon in various materials collected from young infants with proven rubella infection, even though their capacity to respond in normal manner to a challenge with attenuated rubella virus was intact. The authors feel that this represented an inadequate interferon response to the rubella infection. To determine whether interferon might be produced during early course of the infection *in utero*, we have examined tissue homogenates of aborted conceptal materials collected from women with and without clinical rubella. All of the tissues were also examined for the presence of virus. In these studies, the challenge viruses included vesicular stomatitis virus, Sindbis, herpes virus hominis and ECHO 11, and the monitoring cell systems included primary human amnion, human kidney, diploid lung, as well as primary rabbit and monkey kidney cells.

When PHA cultures were pretreated with homogenate uninfected control conceptal materials and challenged with VSV virus, the growth of VSV was actually enhanced when compared to that in control cultures which had not been pretreated. In contrast, when the cultures had been overlayed with rubella-infected placental and fetal tissue homogenates, the cytopathogenic effect and the growth of VSV was delayed for 24 hours or more. Thus, the rubella-infected material appears to contain a material that interferes with the growth of VSV. The characteristics of this material are as follows:

1. It interferes with the growth and development of CPE of certain RNA virus, particularly VSV and Sindbis, but does not effect these same parameters when challenged with herpes virus hominis.

2. It appears to have tissue species specificity.

3. It resists destruction when kept overnight at pH 2.0.

4. It is stable at room temperature and 40°C for many weeks and stable at 56°C for one hour or more.

From this preliminary work, the material present in the rubella-infected conceptal tissue has characteristics similar to interferon.

The interfering activity was found in materials collected from 23 of 40 women who were aborted because of clinical rubella and in materials from only 1 of 10 spontaneous abortions which were not infected by rubella virus. Conceptal materials from 18 of the women with a history of rubella contained virus and materials from 16 or 89 percent of these also contained an interferon-like material. This same type of activity was also present in materials from 27 percent of women with a history of clinical rubella even though virus was not recovered from the abortuses.

These results suggest that the human fetus in the earlier stages of gestation is capable of manufacturing at least small amounts of interferon when infected by rubella virus. Since there are no comparative data the adequacy of this response cannot presently be judged.

Chapter 11

A REVIEW OF THE CURRENT STATUS OF RUBELLA VACCINES

HARRY M. MEYER, JR., PAUL D. PARKMAN, and HOPE E. HOPPS

INTRODUCTION

RUBELLA Virus Vaccine, Live was licensed in the United States in 1969. We are told that 3.4 million doses were released for commercial distribution in the first six months. Presently, new vaccine is being produced at a rate of about two million doses per month; this figure will probably increase more than threefold as additional manufacturers are licensed.

The use of vaccine appears to be progressing relatively smoothly. I say "relatively," since those actually involved in the countless administrative matters attending the beginning of an immunization program might assess the situation somewhat differently. The only significant medical problems coming to our attention thus far have concerned the inadvertent inoculation of pregnant women. While the advisory committees have stressed this contraindication to vaccine use, its occasional occurrence comes as a surprise to no one.

As one proceeds with rubella immunization it is natural and desirable that questions be asked and earlier decisions discussed. Immunization policies like other areas of medical practice should not be static but subject to continuing review and modification when judged appropriate. With this in mind it may be helpful to consider some of the questions pertinent to rubella immunization that have been frequently addressed to us in recent weeks and to discuss the information, new and old, bearing on the subject.

RISK TO FETUS OF ATTENUATED VIRUS

Perhaps the most difficult question to answer concerns the risk to the fetus of the attenuated virus. The results of several small

104

studies involving deliberate vaccination of women scheduled for therapeutic abortion have been previously reported (1-3). Work in this area is continuing but thus far has provided no definite evidence that the attenuated viruses can cross the placenta. The numbers involved are small, however, and for a variety of technical reasons the data fall short of being ideal. It is our impression at present that the attenuated viruses are less likely to infect the fetus but no one is in a position to predict how much less likely.

Anyone hearing of an instance of unintentional inoculation of an expectant mother should certainly make every effort to see that appropriate virus studies are done. The family may decide on therapeutic abortion or on allowing the pregnancy to proceed to term. In either instance the results of laboratory studies could provide useful information regarding the safety of the vaccine.

COMMUNICABILITY OF ATTENUATED VIRUS

Safe use of the vaccine in the general population requires that the attenuated strains be either noncommunicable or incapable of inducing transplacental infection. During our first clinical trials four years ago we found that the vaccine virus could be recovered from the respiratory secretions of most inoculated persons yet these vaccinees were not contagious for intimate contacts (4). These data, when published were supported by other experimental evidence indicating that qualitative and quantitative differences in the performance of the attenuated virus probably accounted for the lack of communicability (4). In the vast clinical experience since 1965 our observations have been confirmed and extended (5). During these vaccine trials protocols were designed to search for evidence of communicability under a variety of conditions favoring intimate contact—sibling to sibling, child to mother and mother to infant as well as institutional settings. Taken as a whole this experience has established the lack of contagiousness of vaccinees for contacts. This is not to say that seroconversion of controls has never occurred. Rarely, contacts have developed antibodies but so infrequently that it has not been possible to incriminate the vaccine. Bear in mind that some background seroconversion due to natural rubella, unintentional vaccination of controls, mislabeling of specimens and laboratory error is to be expected.

One could postulate that pregnant women might be more easily infected and thereby could question the validity of the data collected. Since pregnant individuals have rarely been included as contact controls in vaccine studies one must turn for reassurance to the general epidemiological experience with rubella. We are not aware of information indicating that pregnant women are at increased risk to infection although the evidence does suggest that women in general, if infected are more likely to experience arthritis and other symptoms of disease.

Placing the facts in perspective one cannot deny the theoretical possibility of vaccine virus transmission. However, if the risk is real one can conclude that it must be very slight. The use of all biologics is associated with some degree of risk. Consider for example the potential hazards of vaccination against poliomyelitis, measles and pertussis. In the case of rubella as for these other diseases the various advisory committees have concluded that the risk is negligible in relation to the need and have recommended wide use of the vaccine (6, 7). In weighing relative risks it is well to bear in mind the fact that the presence of *unvaccinated* children in a household constitutes a very clear epidemiological threat to an expectant mother as long as "wild" rubella viruses are circulating in our communities.

VACCINE-INDUCED IMMUNITY AND REINFECTION

To begin the discussion of this question it may be useful to refer to the latest data pertaining to the persistence of rubella antibodies in vaccinated persons. Over the past four years we have conducted eleven rubella vaccine studies at the Arkansas Children's Colony. During the course of this work a variety of attenuated strains of virus have been evaluated (8, 9). Working with these groups it has been possible to obtain a long-term follow-up of these vaccinees for antibody levels. At four years postvaccination the geometric mean titer of hemagglutination-inhibition (HI) antibodies in the first groups given HPV-77 remains stable. We have found a similar pattern of antibody persistence for the other attenuated vaccines although the follow-up period has been shorter.

Having established that these antibodies do persist, let us consider the evidence that antibodies induced by the vaccine, or for that matter by natural rubella, do indeed protect. Protection from clinical disease is easy to demonstrate. Early work by Green and Krugman (10), Plotkin (11), Sever (12), Buescher (13) and Horstmann (14) established that persons with naturally acquired rubella antibodies did not experience clinical symptoms after re-exposure to the virus. In studying an institutional outbreak of epidemic rubella and in reanalyzing some of the Army recruit population sera several years ago Dr. Parkman and I found that persons with naturally acquired antibodies although protected clinically did sometimes have an increase in antibody titer after re-exposure (15). This type of limited reinfection appeared to occur more commonly in persons with low to moderately low pre-existing antibody titer.

The first test of vaccine-induced immunity came three years ago when we challenged 5 girls immunized with HPV-77 8 months to one year earlier (15). These data have been presented many times before. Nevertheless, a review of the information is pertinent to this discussion. In the experiment the 5 previously vaccinated girls and 5 other rubella susceptible girls were inoculated intranasally with 100 $TCID_{50}$ of natural rubella virus. All of the susceptible group experienced a rubella-like illness and developed antibodies. Since none of the previously vaccinated group became ill it was thus established that vaccine-induced antibodies like naturally acquired antibodies could protect against clinical rubella.

The more interesting aspect of the study, however, concerned the results of the virologic testing (15). The unvaccinated girls all shed virus profusely and 4 had demonstrable viremia. Virus was never recovered from the vaccinated group.

Serologic studies were also performed and the results were summarized in the earlier publication (15). Two of the 5 previously vaccinated girls had a boost in preexisting antibody titer after the challenge even though they were not ill and did not shed virus. When we presented the information to the Vaccine Development Board of the NIH in January 1967 we concluded that these two girls had probably experienced a limited reinfection.

Since then several other groups have conducted challenge experiments or have studied vaccinees exposed to natural rubella (5). There have been many variables in these investigations and the type of monitoring has ranged from simple clinical evaluation to detailed virologic examination. In general there has been agreement that any detectable level of antibody seems to afford protection from disease. The debate centers around the significance of subclinical reinfection.

Quite recently we have been involved in a study the results of which touch right at the heart of this matter. Recently rubella was introduced into our population under surveillance at the Arkansas Children's Colony by children exposed at home during Easter vacation. The outbreak at the Colony lasted for about 10 weeks and was monitored by physicians from our laboratory. During this period the physicians were in residence at the Colony and on a daily basis they examined and collected throat swabs from all individuals in cottages where rubella was occurring or suspected. Heparinized blood samples for virus isolation were collected at frequent intervals judged appropriate by the epidemiologic circumstances. Serology specimens were obtained weekly. Perhaps I should mention that the serologic status of all persons at the Colony was already known as a result of our routine surveillance. Since nearly each one of the cottages at the Colony has a mixed population of vaccinees, susceptibles and naturally immune children, we had an ideal situation for direct comparison of the clinical and virologic circumstances associated with primary infection or reinfection.

In all there were 22 primary rubella infections in seronegative persons. With the daily clinical examinations it was possible to detect a rash disease in all of the group. Seventeen vaccinees and approximately 70 naturally immune individuals had a cottage exposure to rubella. None of these evidenced any clinical symptoms suggestive of rubella. Five of the vaccinees and one of the naturally immune children had a significant boost in antibody.

We are interested in directing attention to the preliminary results of virologic studies conducted during the epidemic. Virus was isolated with ease from throat swab specimens collected from unvaccinated persons with natural rubella. In fact the typical case shed virus for between 2 and 3 weeks.

The group with antibodies at the time of exposure as a result of earlier natural infection or earlier vaccination presented a strikingly different picture. Only one of these children shed demonstrable amounts of virus and even here the amount of virus in the throat swab specimens was quite low. One girl who was considered a vaccine failure in that she failed to develop antibodies after vaccination was exposed in this epidemic. Even though she was seronegative she failed to manifest any disease after exposure and shed only a moderate amount of virus.

Collection of specimens for viremia studies poses more of a technical problem. Good sampling, however, was possible on a number of children with classical rubella and on all of the vaccinated persons with evidence of subclinical reinfection. Viremia was demonstrated in each of the unvaccinated, seronegative persons who was studied during the course of the infection. No evidence of viremia was obtained in any of the children with antibodies at the time of exposure or in the "vaccine-failure."

CONCLUSION

As Dr. Stokes mentioned in his keynote speech, there are two important considerations in rubella reinfection: (1) Are successfully vaccinated persons sufficiently resistant to reinfection that one can consider them of no practical consequence in the transmission of rubella? (2) Can we expect protection of the fetus when a girl vaccinated today is exposed to rubella some years hence as a pregnant adult?

Obviously the advisory committees in their prelicensing recommendations felt that the data supported an affirmative answer to both questions, otherwise they would not have endorsed the general vaccination of children as the prime approach to the control of rubella. We think these recent data support the action of the advisory committees and encourage one to feel that the degree of reinfection in rubella is not different from the well documented ability to reinfect recipients of live polio and live measles vaccines. We would also hazard a guess that rubella reinfection will prove to be of no more clinical or epidemiological importance than has been observed in the use of these other live virus vaccines.

In closing we would like to say that we share Dr. Stokes' opinion that natural rubella is less communicable than measles and varicella. For this reason it does seem possible that the vaccination of children against rubella may have a significant effect on herd immunity rather early. If so then rubella may begin to disappear from our communities at a faster rate than was seen with measles during the early phase of that immunization program several years ago. This is an exciting prospect and we hope that it will prove to be true.

REFERENCES

1. Katz, S. L.: Discussion on Sessions III and IV. In International Conference on Rubella Immunization, Bethesda, Maryland, February 18-20, 1969. *Amer. J. Dis. Child.*, 118:317, 1969.
2. Vaheri, A., Vesikari, T., Oker-Blum, N., Seppala, M., Veronelli, J., Robbins, F. C., and Parkman, P.: Transmission of attenuated rubella vaccines to human fetus. A preliminary report. International Conference on Rubella Immunization, Bethesda, Maryland, February 18-20, 1969. *Amer. J. Dis. Child.*, 118:243, 1969.
3. Furukawa, T., Miyata, T., Kondo, K., Kuno, K., Iromura, S., and Takekoshi, T.: Clinical trials of FA 27/3 (Wistar) rubella vaccine in Japan. International Conference on Rubella Immunization, Bethesda, Maryland, February 18-20, 1969. *Amer. J. Dis. Child.*, 118:262, 1969.
4. Meyer, H. M., Jr., Parkman, P. D., and Panos, T. C.: Attenuated rubella virus. II. Production of an experimental live-virus vaccine and clinical trial. *New Eng. J. Med.*, 275:575, 1966.
5. Krugman, S. (Ed.): Proceedings of the International Conference on Rubella Immunization. *Amer. J. Dis. Child.*, 118:1, 1969.
6. Recommendation of the Public Health Service Advisory Committee on Immunization Practices. Morbidity and Mortality Weekly Report. Vol. 18, Number 15, April 12, 1969.
7. Report of the Committee on the Control of Infectious Diseases, American Academy of Pediatrics, Fifteenth Edition, Evanston, Illinois, 1966; Committee Statement, Rubella Virus Vaccine, Newsletter Supplement, April 15, 1969.
8. Meyer, H. M., Jr., Parkman, P. D., Hobbins, T. E., Larson, H. E., Davis, W. J., Simsarian, J. P., and Hopps, H. E.: Attenuated rubella viruses. Laboratory and clinical characteristics. *Amer. J. Dis. Child.*, 118:155, 1969.
9. Meyer, H. M., Jr., Parkman, P. D., and Hopps, H. E.: The control of rubella. *Pediatrics*, 44:5, 1969.
10. Green, R. H., *et al:* Studies of the natural history and prevention of rubella. *Amer. J. Dis. Child.*, 110:348, 1965.

11. Plotkin, S. A., Cornfield, D., and Ingalls, T. H.: Studies of immunization with living rubella virus. *Amer. J. Dis. Child.*, 110:381, 1965.
12. Sever, J. L., Schiff, G. M., and Traub, R. G.: Rubella virus. *JAMA*, 182:663, 1962.
13. Buescher, E. L.: Behavior of rubella virus in adult populations. *Arch. Ges. Virusforsch.*, 16:470, 1965.
14. Horstmann, D. M., *et al:* A natural epidemic of rubella in a closed population: Virologic and epidemiological observations. *Arch. Ges. Virusforsch.*, 16:483, 1965.
15. Meyer, H. M., Jr., Parkman, P. D., Hobbins, T. E., and Ennis, F. A.: Clinical studies with experimental live rubella virus vaccine (Strain HPV-77). *Amer. J. Dis. Child.*, 115:648, 1968.

Chapter 12

INTERPRETATION OF SEROLOGIC FINDINGS FOLLOWING A MASS RUBELLA IMMUNIZATION PROGRAM

R. J. Ferlauto, J. J. McKee, J. F. Pagano, J. A. Gold, K. Graham, and R. Schoengold

INTRODUCTION

R UBELLA, when acquired during pregnancy, has been documented as a major cause of birth defects, including cataracts, deafness, heart defects, micrencephaly and motor and mental retardation. Today, primarily because of the human and economic toll it takes, it is considered a major health problem in the United States. In 1964, the rubella epidemic resulted in thousands of rubella-syndrome children. The exact number will probably never be known, but estimates have gone as high as 40,000. Recently, people at the CDC estimated in dollars and cents the cost of the 1964-1965 rubella epidemic in this country (1). If one assumes a minimum of 10,500 victims and a maximum of 30,000, the direct economic costs alone vary from $539 million to over $1.5 billion; whereas if productivity losses are added to these figures this becomes >840 million to over 2 billion respectively. The development of several rubella vaccines in the past few years promises to prevent such catastrophes from occurring again.

Vaccines have been developed from virus attenuated on green monkey cells (2), human cells (3) and rabbit kidney cells (4). Our involvement has been with the latter, called the "Cendehill" strain.

The Cendehill strain of rubella was first isolated in 1963 by our colleagues at Recherche et Industrie Therapeutique (R.I.T.), Belgium. After primary isolation in monkey kidney cells it was serially passaged in primary rabbit kidney cells for 53 passages. The PRKC substrate was chosen because a unique source of

112

animals was available from a closed colony, free of known pathogens.

We at SK&F have developed this unique vaccine here in the United States and hope to market it in the near future under the name "Cendevax." We have amassed data on over 75,000 vaccinated subjects in the United States and Caribbean area. It is our intention here to discuss some of the information uncovered during this extensive investigation.

SEROLOGICAL ASSAY

The vast majority of all the serological determinations were performed at SK&F Laboratories. It was essential that methodology be perfected whereby large numbers of serum samples could be processed quickly and accurately; therefore a semiautomated microtiter method was developed, using a variation of Stewart's method (*New Eng. J. Med.*, 276:554, 1967). Up to 1,000 serum specimens were tested per day with this method.

The assay involves two equally important phases, as shown in Table 12-I. The serum is first pretreated to remove nonspecific factors, using heat inactivation, kaolin, and pigeon cells. It is then tested with the aid of the Autotiter, an automatic diluting device.

TABLE 12-I

RUBELLA HEMAGGLUTINATION-INHIBITION PROCEDURE

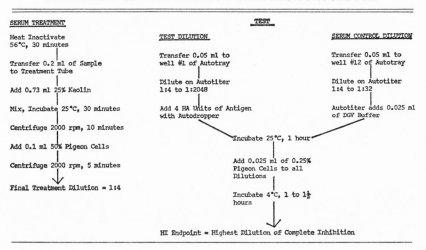

HI Endpoint = Highest Dilution of Complete Inhibition

To process the sera, an array of small laboratory equipment including automatic pipets with disposable tips, large capacity table-top centrifuges which accept disposable test tubes and an automatic dispensing device for addition of kaolin were used.

Because the reagents used in the assay are difficult to standardize, the procedure was monitored with known standard sera. In our experience control sera should comprise approximately 5 percent of the sera being assayed. This level of controls is adequate to detect daily, as well as day to day variation, and more importantly minimizes the chances of error due to improper treatment or dilution of the sera.

This assay should be done by laboratory personnel thoroughly experienced with experimental serological and immunological procedures. Although this mechanization enabled us to process many samples in a short time, we should like to emphasize the need for experienced laboratory personnel in order to monitor the process and interpret the results.

INCIDENCE OF SUSCEPTIBILITY

It has been well documented at recent international meetings that 80 to 90 percent of women of childbearing age are immune to rubella. This level of immunity is usually not reached until the nineteenth year, whereas > 80 percent of preschool children are susceptible to infection. The rate of susceptibility decreases with age, the highest rate of infection occurring between 5 and 10 years (5). In pre-screening populations for rubella immunity, our data, for the most part, mirrors the overall susceptibility picture (Table 12-II). However, we uncovered some exceptions which we feel are of interest and may prove to be of some importance. For example, the degree of immunity in adult females living in "inner city" populations may approach 95%, which is higher than that of their suburban or rural counterparts.

The term "adult" females may delude us concerning the level of protection among females of childbearing age. The 80 to 90 percent immune figure is not achieved until close to 20 years of age; but many women have babies before they reach that age. Therefore, it seemed important to determine how many females older than 13 years are of "childbearing age," and susceptible to rubella.

TABLE 12-II

RUBELLA SUSCEPTIBILITY IN FEMALES OF CHILDBEARING AGE

	13-17 Years		18-35 Years		Total	
Costa Rica	206/85	(41%)	99/25	(25%)	305/110	(36%)
Nassau	181/53	(29%)	13/3	(23%)	194/56	(29%)
Jamaica	933/303	(33%)	17/0		950/303	(32%)
Puerto Rico	85/52	(61%)	449/251	(56%)	534/303	(57%)
California	132/66	(50%)	122/33	(27%)	254/99	(39%)
Colorado	55/5	(9%)	337/33	(10%)	392/38	(10%)
Delaware	309/111	(36%)	13/4	(31%)	322/115	(36%)
Florida	14/4	(29%)	253/78	(31%)	267/82	(31%)
Iowa	0/0		326/43	(13%)	326/43	(13%)
Massachusetts	38/17	(45%)	303/58	(19%)	341/75	(22%)
Minnesota	3/0		100/18	(18%)	103/18	(17%)
Ohio	28/7	(25%)	589/52	(9%)	617/59	(10%)
Pennsylvania	295/67	(23%)	1,260/184	(15%)	1,555/251	(16%)
Wisconsin	85/20	(24%)	233/25	(11%)	318/45	(14%)

Although our overall data show only a 10 to 15 percent susceptibility, there are pockets of high susceptibility. Such obvious pockets in areas where we pre-screened at least 100 females are, for example, Puerto Rico with 57 percent, California (Southern California/San Francisco) with 39 percent, Florida (Gainesville area) with 31 percent, and more underdeveloped areas where much childbearing is done at a younger age, as the country of Costa Rica with 36 percent and the islands of Nassau and Jamaica with 29 percent and 32 percent, respectively.

These findings may be partially explained by the hypothesis that has been made by others that island and rural populations tend to be more susceptible to rubella infection. But this would not explain the situation on the mainland where much of the screening was performed in large urban areas. Such data should make one aware that overall immunity figures that appear in the literature do not in any way guarantee that such will be the case in each and every community.

EFFECTS OF VACCINATION WITH THE CENDEHILL VACCINE

Types of Studies

The clinical evaluation of the Cendehill vaccine was begun in the United States in late 1967 in closed study populations. In these

TABLE 12-III

CENDEHILL VACCINE CLINICAL EVALUATION

Study	No. Centers	No. Participants	% Seroconv.	GMT
Closed	13	664	97.4	1:51
Family	12	1,484	97.6	1:68
Open	13	77,075	97.7	1:72
Adult female	11	906	98.8	1:64

institutionalized groups, rubella-susceptible populations were identified; approximately half were vaccinated and the remainder kept in close daily contact. Six to eight weeks later a second rubella antibody determination was performed. Eighteen such studies were performed by 13 different investigators, involving 664 rubella-susceptible children. In these studies the vaccine was shown to be safe and efficacious with no spread to susceptible contacts; 97.4 percent of the vaccinees seroconverted with a GMT of 1:51, whereas none of the contacts did. Clinical signs and symptoms in the vaccinees were limited to lymphadenopathy in about 10 percent of the subjects. Cendehill virus was isolated in about 50 percent of the attempts.

Family studies were undertaken to test communicability of the vaccine under conditions of more intimate contact. Families were chosen that had two or more rubella-susceptible children (usually preschool) in which the mother was seropositive, or was seronegative but not pregnant and was practicing contraception. Generally, only one of the susceptible children was vaccinated, the others serving as contacts. Twelve such studies were done and the results confirmed what had been established in the closed studies, namely that the vaccine was safe, efficacious and noncommunicable; 97.6 percent of the vaccinees seroconverted with a GMT of 1:68 whereas none of the contacts did.

Thirteen open studies have been completed. These involved over 72,000 individuals, including more than 22,000 susceptibles; ranging in age from six months to 60 years. Concomitantly, over 4,000 subjects were inoculated with saline placebo. In all these studies the incidence of side effects was about the same for both the vaccinated and control populations.

Vaccination of Adult Females

When it became apparent that mature women apparently re-acted differently than children to rubella vaccination with regard to joint symptoms, a series of 11 controlled studies to determine this effect following Cendehill vaccination were carried out in-volving both immune and susceptible individuals given either vac-cine or placebo. Neither the physician nor the individual knew the immune status or the nature of the injection. Over 98 percent of susceptibles seroconverted with a GMT of 1:64.

With regard to the side effects reported (Table 12-IV) from the controlled adult female studies, lymphadenopathy was the only complaint clearly related to Cendehill vaccination. There was a low (not statistically significant) incidence of arthralgia. The arthralgia, when it occurred, was mild and of one to two days duration. This most commonly occurred in the knee or finger joints. There were no recurrences.

It was also of interest to determine whether age had any effect on the immune response to the vaccine, as apparently it does on the side effects experienced. Table 12-V shows the immune re-

TABLE 12-IV

INCIDENCE OF "SIDE EFFECTS" REPORTED IN PLACEBO-CONTROLLED DOUBLE-BLIND STUDIES IN ADULT WOMEN

	Vaccinees		Placebos	
	Seronegative (115)	Seropositive (113)	Seronegative (106)	Seropositive (125)
Arthralgia	9 (7.8%)†	5 (4.4%)	4 (3.8%)	5 (4.0%)
Arthritis	2 (1.7%)	1 (0.9%)	1 (0.9%)	0
Lymphadenopathy	38 (33.0%)	15 (13.3%)	13 (12.3%)	11 (8.8%)
Temperature elevation	8 (7.0%)	12 (10.6%)	8 (7.6%)	8 (6.4%)
Rash	10 (8.7%)	7 (6.2%)	2 (1.9%)	10 (8.0%)
Local reaction	4 (3.5%)	3 (2.7%)	1 (0.9%)	2 (1.6%)
Myalgia	6 (5.2%)	7 (6.2%)	1 (0.9%)	1 (0.8%)
U.R.I.	27 (23.5%)	36 (31.9%)	23 (21.7%)	16 (12.8%)
G.I. upset	7 (6.1%)	5 (4.4%)	8 (7.6%)	6 (4.8%)
Miscellaneous*	12 (10.4%)	8 (7.1%)	6 (5.7%)	8 (6.4%)

* Includes headache, "fever blister," vertigo, "menstrual problems," etc.

† Includes a vaccinee who failed to seroconvert; therefore reported reaction probably not due to the vaccine. The correct incidence of arthralgia is actually 7.0%.

TABLE 12-V

AGE VS. IMMUNE RESPONSE IN SUSCEPTIBLE FEMALE VACCINEES

Age Range	Number	No. Converted	Percentage Conversion	GMT°
6 and less	3,340	3,362	98.0	86.5
7-13	5,113	5,009	97.9	72.9
14-17	318	314	98.7	63.4
18-21	265	259	97.7	59.6
22-25	63	61	96.9	40.6
26-29	37	36	97.5	42.7
30-33	15	15	100	38.5
34-37	9	9	100	43.5
38-42	9	8	83.4	45.2
>42	5	4	80.0	107.6

° Non-converters not included in calculation.

sponse in susceptible, vaccinated females. There is no apparent difference with age.

Vaccination of Immune Individuals

In any vaccination program, whether publically sponsored or not, the vast majority of subjects are already immune to rubella. Yet this immune status is unknown to the physician and, for the most part, to the individual also. Patient history has been shown many times to be an unreliable index of past infection. What

TABLE 12-VI

BOOSTER EFFECT° OF RUBELLA VACCINATION

Prevaccination Titer	No.	Decrease	Postvaccination Titer No Change	Increase
1:8	19	0	8 (42%)	11 (58%)
1:16	41	0	22 (54%)	19 (46%)
1:32	64	0	41 (64%)	23 (36%)
1:64	125	1	106 (85%)	18 (14%)
1:128	267	6 (2%)	238 (89%)	23 (9%)
1:256	367	17 (5%)	327 (89%)	23 (6%)
1:512	261	27 (10%)	227 (87%)	7 (3%)
1:1,024	125	20 (16%)	105 (84%)	0
1:2,048	12	5 (41%)	7 (58%)	0
Total	1,281	76 (6%)	1,081 (84%)	124 (10%)

° Booster effect = fourfold or greater change.

then are the effects of Cendehill rubella vaccination on persons who are already immune? Table 12-VI illustrates the effect of immunization on existing rubella antibody.

These data permitted analysis of age and sex distribution, but the only significant finding seems to be that of those individuals with a pre-existing titer below 1:64, 43 percent responded with a significant booster effect (fourfold or greater), regardless of sex or age, whereas of those with a titer of 1:64 or greater only 6 percent showed a boost response.

It is of interest to note that vaccination of immune individuals did not cause any unusual side effects. There was no significant difference between saline and vaccine inoculated immune individuals.

Time of Antibody Appearance after Vaccination

In many situations it is important to both patient and physician to know how soon after vaccination a susceptible individual develops an anti-rubella titer. It is not feasible to obtain such data from single individuals because of the necessity of frequent blood samplings. Most data of this type reflect not the appearance of antibody but rather the time when the investigator looked for antibody. The data in Table 12-VII represent a pooling of all information collected in our studies on individuals bled soon after vaccination and up to 40 days later. We know from our closed studies that over 95 percent of the susceptible population had responded with a specific antibody titer by six weeks. The

TABLE 12-VII

APPEARANCE OF SPECIFIC RUBELLA ANTIBODY FOLLOWING
CENDEHILL VACCINATION

Postvaccination Days	No.	No.	Conversion %	GMT
0-4	11	4	35	1:20
5-9	13	6	46	1:45
10-14	71	21	30	1:25
15-19	18	10	56	1:17
20-24	26	25	96	1:42
25-29	75	73	97	1:42
30-34	3	3	100	1:64
35-39	31	29	94	1:54

apparent appearance of antibody in a few individuals in less than ten days should be interpreted with some caution. There is a likelihood, supported by the low level of antibody detected, that these persons may have had a low level of preexisting antibody and erronously had been designated susceptible, prior to vaccination. The one conclusion that these data do seem to support is the fact most people have seroconverted by 30 days, although indeed they may not have reached their peak antibody titers by that time.

Challenge Studies

Attempts were made to challenge persons previously immunized with Cendehill vaccine in an attempt to determine its protective effect. Table 12-VIII illustrates the results of two separate challenge studies with 10^4TCID50 of wild rubella Brown strain. Although virus was recovered from the nasopharynx three out of five times, there were no signs or symptoms of rubella infection in any of the vaccinees, although nonimmune challenged individuals did develop typical rubella. Furthermore, there were some susceptible contracts exposed to these immune-challenged individuals and no virus was spread to them. It is difficult to draw any conclusion from such a small sample, but it does seem as if the level of the antibody titer may determine both the booster effect (as we have already shown) as well as viral replication in the nasopharynx. Apparently this replicating virus is noncommunicable. More data is needed to clarify these points.

Duration of Antibody

Does the Cendehill vaccine impart a lasting immunity? It will take many years before such data are available. However, from

TABLE 12-VIII

WILD VIRUS CHALLENGE OF CENDEHILL VACCINEES

Subject	Time Since Vaccination	Titer at Challenge	Titer Post-challenge	Virus Isolate
PA23	18 months	1:160	1:160	No
PA54	18 months	1:160	1:80	No
PA41	18 months	1:20	1:160	Yes
PA46	18 months	1:20	1:320	Yes
B68682	219 days	1:16	1:128	Yes

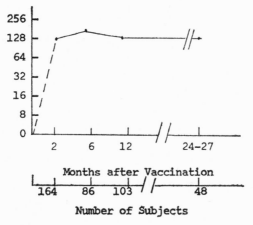

Figure 12-1. Duration of antibody.

what is available, primarily from the early studies in Europe (Fig. 12-1), it would seem that the titers do not decrease appreciably in the more than two years they have been followed. This situation seems to be about the same as the three studies in the United States where we have one-year data.

Fetal Studies

The rationale for developing a rubella vaccine is to protect the unborn child from the ravages of an infection in a susceptible mother. The use of the rubella vaccine in children will probably

TABLE 12-IX

FETAL ABORTION STUDIES

Center	Subject	Age	Wks. Preg. at Vacc.	Aborted Postvacc.	HI Titer at Vacc.	HI Titer at Abort.	Later Serum*	Fetal Virus Recovery
Switzerland ..	RO	22	10	18 days	<8	256		none
Switzerland ..	PI	25	4	20 days	<8	32		none
Switzerland ..	BO	28	7	36 days	<8	64		none
Japan	A-1	29	9	17 days	8	8	16	none
Japan	A-2	19	7	19 days	8	16	128	none
Japan	A-3	28	6	17 days	<8	8	32	none
Japan	A-6	27	7	16 days	<8	<8	16	none
Japan	A-7	29	7	17 days	8	8	32	none

* 4-6 weeks after vaccination.

eventually eliminate susceptible mothers. However, in the intervening years there will be many women of childbearing age who will want the assurance of protection that vaccination will give them. The official government recommendations for the use of rubella vaccine cautions against their use in women, since no one knows the effect of attenuated strains of rubella on the fetus. Some data from overseas is available in which rubella-susceptible women who were candidates for therapeutic abortions were vaccinated, and the products of conception examined for virus. Table 12-IX shows that a total of 8 women who had no titer (or minimal) were vaccinated during the fourth and tenth week of pregnancy. They were aborted 16 to 36 days later. All had boosts in titer either at the time of abortion or within four to six weeks of vaccination. No virus was recovered from the fetal material.

SUMMARY AND CONCLUSIONS

We have presented data based on serologic findings following extensive immunization studies with Cendehill rubella vaccine in over 70,000 individuals. In closed, family, adult female, and open studies the vaccine was shown to be efficacious, causing a seroconversion in over 95 percent of the individuals inoculated; noncommunicable, and safe, with occasional lymphadenopathy the only real vaccine-related side effect. We feel these data support our claim that the Cendehill vaccine provides the means of eradicating rubella and the consequences of its fetal infections in the near future.

REFERENCES

1. Shavell, Stephen: Costs of the 1964-1965 rubella epidemic. *6th Annual Immunization Conference*, March 11-13, 1969, Atlanta, Georgia.
2. Parkman, P. D., Meyer, H. M., Jr., and Hopps, H. E.: Production and laboratory testing of experimental live rubella virus vaccine. *International Symposium on Rubella Vaccine*, London, 1968, *Sym. Series Immunobiol. Standard*, 11:261-70, 1969, Karger, Basel.
3. Plotkin, S. A.: Development of RA 27/3 attenuated rubella virus grown in WI-38 cells. *Ibid*, 11:249-260, 1969.
4. Huygelen, C., Peetermans, J., Colinet, G., Zygraich, N., and Fagard, P.: Production and safety testing of live rubella virus vaccine (Cendehill strain). *Ibid*, 11:229-36, 1969.
5. Sencer, D. J., Witte, J. J., and Karchmer, A. W.: The epidemiology of rubella in the United States. *Ibid*, 11:9-14, 1969.

Chapter 13

OBSTETRIC PROBLEMS ASSOCIATED WITH RUBELLA

ALFRED L. KALODNER

R UBELLA is a common communicable disease of childhood characterized by mild constitutional symptoms. The rash is similar to mild measles or mild scarlet fever, or a combination of both, and there is a marked enlargement and tenderness of the postoccipital, retro-auricular, and posterior cervical lymph nodes. In general, rubella may be considered as the least dangerous of all of the acute communicable diseases of childhood. Under ordinary circumstances, there are few complications and the signs and symptoms subside as rapidly as they appear (1).

With the disease thus defined and described, what has caused rubella to take on increasing significance, and why has so much effort been expended in eradication of this "least dangerous of all the acute communicable diseases in childhood"? First, clinical observation has revealed that although rubella is primarily a disease of childhood, it does strike adults; and although it is generally a mild disease in childhood, when it does strike adults, especially postpubertal females, there are increasing evidences of arthritis, arthralgia, and occasionally encephalitis. Secondly, following the initial observations of Gregg in Australia (2) demonstrating the high incidence of cataracts in children born to mothers who contracted the disease early in pregnancy, numerous additional observations of other congenital defects have been reported by various authors (3-9). The clinical observations and reports of these abnormalities have gained increasing significance as obstetrics has moved from the archaic art of accouchement to a more modern approach of human growth and development with an increasing importance of neonatology—a combined area of obstetrics and pediatrics.

No longer is it acceptable to present to the pediatrician for newborn care, a baby damaged or compromised by disease, constitutional factors, inadequate prenatal care or other factors yet unidentified, but open to research, identification and correction. A case in point is the disease now under discussion—rubella. Prior to 1941 and Gregg's observations, nothing was known of the importance of rubella and its damaging effects on the fetus when contracted during early pregnancy. Clinical observation followed, with the identification of the "rubella syndrome," and following the 1963-1964 rubella epidemic in the United States, the "expanded rubella syndrome" was outlined (10).

Rubella Syndrome:

1. Hearing loss in one or both ears and of varying degree. Often it is not detected at birth and sometimes not until a child reaches school age.

2. Eye defects, most commonly described of which are cataracts, glaucoma, unusually small size of the eyeball, lesions of the retina, and clouding of the cornea not associated with glaucoma.

3. Heart defects, which also may not be apparent at birth.

4. Anomalies of the central nervous system, the most common of which are abnormally small size of the head and mental retardation.

Expanded Rubella Syndrome:

1. Small size at birth despite a full-term pregnancy, many of these infants weigh less than 5 pounds at birth. An infant born at term weighing 2 pounds 2 ounces was reported. Many of these infants have feeding problems and gain weight slowly. Diarrhea also occurs with some frequency in these infants.

2. Bleeding tendency associated with low blood platelets, known as thrombocytopenic purpura. This is generally manifested in these infants as reddish or purplish spots scattered over the entire body, particularly over the face. Some infants on blood test are found to have abnormally low blood platelets but present no external evidence of a bleeding tendency.

3. Enlarged liver and spleen.

4. Jaundice, caused by excessive bile pigments in the blood, and manifested as yellowish discoloration of the skin and white part of the eyeball.

5. Swollen lymph nodes. A single node, or many nodes in different parts of the body may be involved.

6. Hepatitis, or inflammation of the liver.

7. Lesions which involve bones of the arms and legs, detectable only by x-ray.

8. Anemia and occasionally low white blood cell count.

9. Pneumonia.

10. Encephalitis and meningitis, usually indicated by a full fontanel, abnormal spinal fluid, irritability, convulsions and other symptoms.

11. Injury to the heart muscle evidenced by symptoms of heart failure and abnormal electrocardiographic tracings.

12. Abnormal fingerprints, palmar creases and other skin patterns.

13. Other congenital malformations and lesions.

To further emphasize the severe damage caused by this disease when associated with early pregnancy, studies have shown that there was an increase of 50 percent in the spontaneous fetal death rate above those expected in a control group of similar patients (11).

Investigation has revealed that not only does the rubella virus cause a higher incidence of spontaneous fetal death, the "rubella syndrome," the "expanded rubella syndrome," but also in normal newborn infants born of infected mothers there is a continuous shedding of live virus for six months (and possibly longer) which presents a problem in the care of affected newborns. Infants with congenital rubella are capable of spreading the infection.

The severe risk to the fetus caused by rubella during early pregnancy has been reported variously as ranging from 15 percent to a high of 50 percent. The last epidemic in the United States in 1963-1964 resulted in an estimated 50,000 abnormal pregnancies and about 20,000 infants with severe birth defects.

All the reports of birth defects occurring in the literature starting with Gregg in 1941 until the "Great Outbreak" in 1964 were just so much didactic information. Positive confirmatory diagnosis of the disease rubella was lacking—rather it was based on clinical impression and symptomatology. Subclinical infection, whether natural or induced by the widespread use of immune globulin resulted in further clouding of the diagnostic picture.

A positive diagnosis could only be made by actually isolating the rubella virus or by blood testing for rubella antibody titer. Since 1964, specific laboratory tests have been developed which enable the physician to not only confirm rubella infection but also to detect immunity years after infection. The development of a live rubella virus vaccine in 1966 was the next step in the logical order of control—recognition of a disease; positive diagnosis of the disease; specific prevention of the disease and finally eradication of the problem. Finally, an answer seemed to be in the immediate offing.

Compared to the hectic days of the 1963-1964 epidemic, when all obstetricians were inundated with requests for immune globulin, when therapeutic abortion became the major consideration of the hospital staff (whether for actual or imagined rubella) and when obstetricians were caught with their therapeutic armamentarium down—the present-day problems presented by the arrival of the vaccine are minimal. However, minimal though they may be, answers are needed, proper management is dictated, and further refinements are necessitated before we may rest on our laurels for the eradication of one problem in the ever-expanding sphere of human growth and development.

Currently, therefore, the following problems present to the obstetrician-pediatrician-neonatologist:

1. The proper age-group for the administration of the vaccine.

2. The development of a vaccine for the use in the "high-risk adult."

3. The implications of improperly given vaccination.

Much has been written and said regarding the proper "priority groups" to be given the vaccine. Should it be the 5- to 9-year-old over a period of two to three years as advised by the Public Health Service? Should it be the susceptible postpartal female? It is obvious that by whatever means priority groups are established, problems will occur in the "high-risk female" i.e. the schoolteacher, etc.

It should be evident at this time that the hemagglutination-inhibition test (HI), despite its susceptibility to error, should be made a standard prenatal blood test. If for no other reason than allaying the fear in the pregnant woman regarding the possibility of her contracting the disease and damaging her baby. It is interesting to note that my own experience with the HI testing has revealed that of 286 patients tested—70 or 28 percent had an HI titer of less than 1:10, and hence are adjudged susceptible to rubella. Historically, 31 percent of those who gave history of disease had less than 1:10 and 24 percent who stated that they did not have the disease had an HI titer over 1:20.

The development of a vaccine that can be safely given to pregnant women is a high priority, since the possibility of vaccinating all potential victims is extremely small. More important, more information is needed regarding the present vaccine, HVP-77, as to its potential for placental transfer, its potential for cross-vaccination, and the seriousness of the side effects when given to adults. Further investigation should be carried out in the use of the Cendehill strain, which has reportedly not been isolated from the products of conception.

I can only state personally, that until such a vaccine is developed, all pregnant patients should be tested for susceptibility; those that are HI negative should be vaccinated in the immediate postpartum period when the chances for conception are extremely low, when the desire for conception control are extremely high, and when the pregnant state (post-pregnant would better describe the time) offers some protection from the arthralgia and arthritic side-effect complaints of vaccination in adults.

Finally, a new complication presents itself for management—iatrogenic threat to the health of the conceptus. Improperly administered vaccine, such as vaccinating postpubertal females without thought to the possibility of pregnancy or pregnancy control can result in production of the rubella syndrome. It cannot be stated strongly enough—if a postpubertal female is to be vaccinated, special care should be taken: (1) test for immunity (HI); (2) pregnancy test; (3) prescription of a medically acceptable method of contraception; (4) full disclosure of the risks involved if she should become pregnant; (5) obtain a written, informed consent; (6) finally, DON'T GIVE IT.

REFERENCES

1. Nelson, Waldo E.: *Textbook of Pediatrics*. Philadelphia, W. B. Saunders.
2. Gregg, N. M.: Congenital cataracts following German measles in the mother. *TR. Ophth. Soc. Australia*, 3:35, 1941.
3. Avery, G. B., *et al:* Rubella syndrome after inapparent maternal illness. *Am. J. Dis. Child.*, 110:444, 1965.
4. Brown, G. C.: Consequences of natural exposure to rubella during pregnancy. *Proc. Soc. Exp. Biol. Med.*, 127:340, 1968.
5. Heggie, A. D.: Rubella: current concepts in epidemiology and teratology. *Ped. Clin. N. Am.* 13:251, 1966.
6. Horstmann, D. M.: 1st trimester exposure to rubella. *JAMA*, 204:1153, 1968.
7. Lundstrom, R.: Rubella during pregnancy. *Acta Paediat. (Stockholm)*, Supp. 133, 1962.
8. Sever, J. L., *et al:* Rubella epidemic, 1964. Effect on 6,000 pregnancies. *Am. J. Dis. Child.*, 110:395, 1965.
9. Siegel, M., *et al:* Fetal mortality in maternal rubella: Results in a prospective study from 1957 to 1964. *Am. J. Obstet. Gynec.*, 96:247, 1966.
10. Rubella. U. S. Dept. HEW Children's Bur. Jane S. Lin-Fu, Ped. Cons. Div. of Health Serv., Children's Bureau.
11. Burrows, S., and Bollman, C.: Rubella HI test in obstetric population. *Obstet. Gynec.*, 33:703, 1969.
12. Deibel, R., Cohen, S. M., and Ducharme, C. P.: Serology of rubella: Virus neutralization, immunofluorescence in BHK 21 cells, and hemagglutination-inhibition. *N. Y. J. Med.*, 68:1355, 1968.
13. Michael, R. H., and Medearis, D. N., Jr.: A new antibody test for rubella. *Pediatrics*, 40:787, 1967.
14. Rauls, W. E., *et al:* Serologic diagnosis and fetal involvement in maternal rubella. *JAMA*, 203:627, 1968.
15. Sever, J. L., *et al:* Frequency of rubella antibody titre among pregnant women and other human and animal populations. *Obstet. Gynec.*, 23:153-159, 1964.
16. Skinner, W. E.: Routine rubella antibody titre determinations in pregnancy. *Obstet. Gynec.*, 33:301, 1969.
17. Hilleman, M. R.: Toward prophylaxis of prenatal infection by viruses. *Obstet. Gynec.*, 33:461, 1969.
18. Stawarz, G. L., *et al:* Rubella—virus hemagglutination-inhibition test. *New Eng. J. Med.*, 276:554, 1967.

Chapter 14

LEGAL RESPONSIBILITIES OF LABORATORIES IN THERAPEUTIC ABORTION

CYRIL H. WECHT

THE matter of legal responsibility for laboratories in the whole area of therapeutic abortion, of course, is nowhere near as great a problem and threat as it is for the clinician. Nevertheless, a significant degree of responsibility does exist. Therapeutic abortion raises many real problems today. Of course, it becomes mired down in moral technological problems which makes it difficult to discuss in a candid and relatively objective fashion. The problem is that everyone has his own views and strong feelings which really are not based as much on science as they are on deeply, deeply rooted theological and philosophical training. The question of therapeutic abortion, which really is so germane to the subject of this conference, is one that physicians in this country should consider in great detail. I think there are not many physicians who appreciate the fact that in Pennsylvania, for example, there really is no legal basis upon which a therapeutic abortion can be performed. One can even question in a strict, technical sense whether in the State of Pennsylvania, a therapeutic abortion can be done legally even to save the life of the mother. Of course, we all know that therapeutic abortions have been done and are being done in increasing numbers, but the fact is that anywhere from two-thirds to three-fourths or more of therapeutic abortions being done in Pennsylvania are obviously and clearly in violation of the existing law.

My own views on the subject of abortion fall very clearly into the so-called liberal line, but something offends me always about hypocrisy whether it be on the part of physicians, attorneys or legislators in my own jurisdiction, I think that the ones who have been most lax and faulty are the legislators who have avoid-

129

ed the promulgation of adequate and modern legislation. I would like to hear from a physician, particularly one who is cloaked in the immunity of the academic world who has nothing to fear, who has tenure and so on, who is not advocating some change in the Pennsylvania law. Physicians in California were willing to be delicensed; they were willing to go to jail over this matter. The professor and chairman of the Department of Obstetrics in New Haven at Yale University was willing to go to jail to carry his case to the Supreme Court on the matter of contraceptive information, which as you know in Massachusetts and Connecticut cannot be given out legally. I toss the challenge out to physicians—now is your time to become Pennsylvania's hero (or in whatever jurisdiction that is similarly in need of legal redress). You can carry the battle and you do not have to worry about being elected to anything.

A case of exposure to rubella does provide specific and just cause to terminate a pregnancy. This does not, it must be remembered, constitute a legal justification for performing the procedure. Now then, the responsibility obviously lies on the shoulders of the people in the laboratories and ultimately in the primary instance on the shoulders of the obstetricians to make a determination as to whether or not an abortion should be performed. Dr. Kalodner cited some statistics and figures as to the incidence of the rubella syndrome in the newborn in women who have been exposed to the disease in the first trimester of pregnancy. The statistics seem to vary a little bit but I think the minimum figure that I have seen is 20 to 25 percent of infants born to women who have been exposed to rubella in the first trimester of pregnancy will show some phase of the rubella syndrome. How severe it will be is questionable and some statistics go much higher. I saw an article recently that 58 percent of such children will have some kind of a hearing defect. Now this is a serious problem and a woman has a right to be informed of this difficulty and she has a right to make a final determination with all information whether or not her pregnancy will continue. I believe that a physician is ethically and morally remiss no matter what his own religion and philosophical tenets may be if he does not call it to the attention of the woman.

Strange as it might seem to some of us in the field, I daresay that there are millions and millions of women of the childbearing age and millions of women who do become pregnant who do not know about German measles, who do not know about what this means in terms of defects and real tragedy to the youngsters when they are born seven, eight or nine months later. So the burden for proper and complete communication then in a very real sense, not only legally but morally and ethically, falls upon the physician.

There are several situations in which the laboratory assumes a significant degree of responsibility concerning the accurate diagnosis of rubella. Let us say that you are asked to check for pregnancy and you say that there is a pregnancy based upon your test and in fact, there is not a pregnancy, a false positive and on the basis of this information, the physician then decides that this woman should not be given the vaccine. Then it is found out later that she was not pregnant and subsequently does become pregnant and the child is born with some kind of a defect. Obviously, then, there could well be the basis for a malpractice action against the physician and against the laboratory. Whether or not one could prove, and of course one really could not prove in a test tube sense the teratogenic defect being associated with the exposure to rubella, in the eyes of the law there could well be such proof given.

An analogy to this could be in the cases that have recently come down, a few over a million dollars in value and some between a half million and a million dollars relative to the use of quadruple vaccines where people have wound up with permanent vegetative states. Did this come about because of a reaction to the quadruple vaccine or was it due to something else, just a natural occurring disease process. Well, this would be a question to be answered by the judge and the jury. No scientist can answer unequivocally yes or no, although some people foolishly from time to time will attempt to do so, becoming very wrapped up in the adversary proceedings. This is an extremely dangerous thing to do on the witness stand.

Now let us say that you give a false negative laboratory test and the woman is really pregnant and the doctor then, on the basis of

your negative pregnancy test does give the woman the vaccine
and she goes on to give birth to a child who has some kind of defect which can be associated with the rubella syndrome. Obviously then you would also have liability in such an instance. The
same thing would be true with regard to the rubella antibody
testing. If a test shows a high or a significant antibody titer and
on the basis of that, the obstetrician does not give the vaccine and
it is later discovered that this test was erroneous and the woman subsequently goes on to give birth to a child with defects,
then there is the basis for liability assuming again that a child is
born with such problems.

Let us say that you do the antibody testing and report that
there is not a significant titer and on the basis of this, the physician gives the vaccine. The test is incorrect and the woman was
pregnant; presume she goes on to give birth to a child that has
defects that could fall into the rubella syndrome, possibly due to
transplacental passage of the virus. You could then be liable
again. In regard to this subject, sufficient data are not yet available, although studies are being done in Japan and in Finland in
which women who have decided to have a therapeutic abortion
are being given the vaccine at periodic intervals and then the
products of conception are being studied virologically. This
may provide adequate data regarding passage of vaccine virus.

Also, the laboratory must be concerned about what kind of
tests are done. As you know, some of the tests are not indicated in certain instances. It is my understanding that the antibody titers which developed as a result of the vaccine cannot be
adequately tested for with immunofluoresence tests and not
very well with complement-fixation. Antibodies developed as
a result of vaccination should be determined by use of the hemagglutination-inhibition test. Then if you want to check for
titers later on and determine whether subsequent levels are from
vaccine or natural exposure, you must select the proper test. So
you must understand the immunologic and serologic sequelae to
immunization and natural exposure in order to provide competent testing.

Now then, there are some things which are common denominators in anything we do in the laboratory and which are as ap-

plicable in this field as they would be in any other field of testing, i.e., basic hematology, bacteriology, and so on. These relate to the training of people, the kind of equipment used, test materials (e.g. controls), and selection and condition of clinical specimens. Unless statutory provisions apply, things are left very much up in the air. Let us say that a laboratory becomes involved in one of the hypothetical malpractice situations that I have just posed to you. Lest everyone become fearful and hostile to the law, let us put the law aside for a moment and consider this question. What is your responsibility as laboratory directors, physicians, and administrators? Is it to try and make the correct diagnoses? Of primary importance is that the laboratory personnel are properly trained. If there is no confidence of your own capability, refer them somewhere else. I think there is a tendency on the part of too many laboratories to jump into too many kinds of testing procedures without proper background, and you can be assured that in these cases which would fall generally into a field of legal liability, the attorneys who handle these cases for the most part are very well trained and competent. They can ask a "million questions" which are pertinent and they will determine and evaluate specific training of technologists performing tests and details of their study programs, what kind of unknowns and control samples were used, were results reviewed by laboratory directors, and a myriad of other factors.

Everybody becomes extremely bitter when they become the object or the subject of a malpractice action. This is understandable, particularly when an action is unjustified, although the definition of an unjustified malpractice action obviously leaves much in the area of discussion. In cases where someone has been harmed, it is, simply, a matter of who is to pay and in what way. Nobody wants to put the physician or laboratory director in jail. These are not criminal actions and at the same time, nobody is going to turn away and say it is alright because you have saved "x" number of lives, you are entitled to "x" number of goofs during the rest of your professional career. If you are driving home this afternoon and you go through a red light and kill somebody, you can show all the merit badges you have from your local mayor and the state police for thirty years of absolute, wonderful driving in which you have never even gotten a traffic ticket, and that is not going to make a darn bit of difference to the person you have just killed or maimed. This is what it is all about. There is something more basic to this than your fear of or adherence to the laws, which is your adherence to what is good medicine and laboratory practice. What is good medicine and laboratory practice, I assure you, will always be good law.

In summation, I would say to you first, if you are going to get into this business of rubella testing, then you owe a responsibility (1) to the patients, (2) to the physicians who use your laboratory, and (3) to yourself. I would put them in that order incidentally. You owe a responsibility to see to it that you know what this test is all about, to read as much about it, and if necessary to take courses in the subject. You must be sure that technicians who work in your laboratory are properly trained in this field.

Once the test is offered, a primary important factor is to obtain a proper history on each case. You must have adequate ground on each case in order to select proper testing procedures. Such factors as the time of exposure, whether patient is pregnant, etc. will determine the proper testing procedure to be used. What about other infectious diseases that might be interfering with results of rubella tests? All these things are matters for you to discuss if necessary with the referring physician. Then, be certain that the test procedure has an adequate system of quality control.

As you know, the incidence of malpractice actions involving pathologists and laboratories is much, much lower than it is with regard to clinicians, particularly certain kinds of clinicians and it is lower than one finds with radiologists. Anesthesiologists, of course have a high incidence, almost as high as some surgical specialties. So comparatively, you do not have to be so terribly afraid of legal action but you must consider the fact that you could be indirectly putting the clinician into jeopardy because of shoddy laboratory procedures. The law places a much greater burden upon medical science in the pharmaceutical industries and upon everybody involved in those instances in which a particular medication, a particular surgical practice, a particular routine, or anything that has not yet been fully established and universally accepted as routine. The further you are away from universal acceptance and complete uniform adherence to a recognized kind of procedure, the more you move back towards something which is experimental. And as you move back towards the experimental field, your legal responsibility becomes that much greater.

Time does not permit me to go into informed consent. I think you all have a pretty good idea of what it is. I will simply emphasize the importance of having things in writing. Do not ever be so busy or so bored or indifferent that you do not take a few minutes to write things. This is always a good procedure to follow when you speak with the doctor and obtain information from him. Also, when you give him information that is not contained on the reporting sheet, make sure that anything said is salient, and also that anything controversial or in which anything that is a significant difference of scientific opinion is so indicated. Also, be sure that such information is germane to the therapy that is to be undertaken or withheld on the basis of your laboratory tests. And all of such discussion should be recorded. That will be your best defense, if defense is justified. The more that is not written, the more susceptible you are to all kinds of inferences being drawn, to all kinds of innuendos being raised in a subsequent action, unjustified as they may be.

I hope that I have not frightened you; I do not mean to suggest that there is going to be a rash of malpractice actions relating to rubella. Most laboratories are able to handle pregnancy tests and most laboratories who get into this field will be able to handle the antibody titer determination for rubella. If one instance of faulty testing does occur, that is perhaps one too many, not because of legal implication, but because that one could result in the birth of a youngster with serious defects and tremendous emotional pain and suffering for the family.

Chapter 15

MANDATORY REQUIREMENTS FOR RUBELLA SEROLOGIC TESTING

ROBERT A. MacCready and JOAN B. DANIELS

MANDATORY requirements for serologic testing resolves it-self into two major questions. The first question consists of the pro and con of having legislation enacted that would make rubella testing mandatory in women as a premarital requirement or even earlier. The second question, on the other hand, is concerned with the necessity of having mandatory requirements in the technique and management of the rubella immunity tests that are performed, usually the hemagglutination-inhibition (HI) test, whether or not the rubella testing itself is a mandatory procedure. These questions are important matters of public health policy.

As indicated, the first question involves a discussion of the pro and con of mandatory testing for rubella antibody. Indeed the aim of a bill—not passed—in an earlier Massachusetts Legislature was the testing for rubella susceptibility as a requirement in all women about to be married. The purpose at least of such a requirement is laudable on the premise that the required testing, followed by prompt vaccination of the women found susceptible along with measures to postpone pregnancy, would indeed reduce greatly the fetal wastage and disastrous abnormalities resulting from rubella contracted in the early part of pregnancy. These very important concerns can hardly be overstated, especially with another rubella outbreak predicted in a year or so.

Actually in this complex problem there are a number of reasons for reluctance in favoring mandatory testing. To begin with, even on a voluntary, selective basis public health and other virology laboratories are already hard-pressed to meet the current demand. Consequently they would find it difficult or impossible to meet adequately the very large increase that would be imposed by a blanket, mandatory regulation for rubella antibody testing.

136

The Massachusetts Public Health Virus Laboratory, for example, is now performing HI tests at the rate of about 5,000 per year with one virologist and two technicians, a rate that is already expected to increase to 30,000 during the year without mandatory requirements.

Moreover the vast majority of the mothers of the approximately 100,000 babies born in a given year in Massachusetts would not be covered by premarital testing done that year. Thus in a mandatory premarital program the very population now most in need of the service—the mothers who have been married for some time—would not be served. Mandatory testing at an earlier age, for example fourteen, also would miss the population of mothers immediately concerned. There is, in any case, the very real risk that too great a load—always with the too few trained people available—will impose such a burden that adequate response can be achieved only by an unfortunate competition jeopardizing other important responsibilities of the modern public health laboratory.

The rather inevitable result, in fact, of this overdemand, since it could not be met adequately in so many areas by the existing public health and other competent virus laboratories, would be the rather prompt stimulation of rubella antibody testing by a distressing number of laboratories not equipped with the experience and know-how for virology laboratory work. Clearly we have no quarrel with the potentialities of a number of virus laboratories which, though not now performing diagnostic rubella testing, have capabilities to perform the test completely. We do, however, fear the performance of the HI test by the many laboratory workers and others who are not trained and experienced in diagnostic virology. However well-assembled and standardized a commercial test kit for the HI test may be, and therefore "easy" to use correctly, it is also easy to use incorrectly, especially by any but an experienced virology serologist. With the tremendous number of tests that would have to be done if mandatory testing became a reality, can we not in fact predict invasion into the field by opportunists and others, who are just not equipped to do the reliable work so necessary if disasters from inaccurate laboratory reports are not otherwise to follow?

Further, we find troubling the inevitable inflexibility of any

laws passed now requiring mandatory testing for rubella antibodies, when even a few years of widespread use of the new rubella vaccine may so reduce the number of nonimmune women
that a much more selective testing for rubella immunity may
later be deemed adequate. Indeed, should later studies reveal
that a pregnant woman can be vaccinated without hazard to the
fetus, and we are *not* predicting this, might it not then be simpler and more economical to immunize without laboratory tests
for susceptibility women not previously vaccinated? Even now it
is argued that available public health monies might be spent more
usefully on more extensive and aggressive vaccination programs
for the children that should be vaccinated than to encumber the
significant expenditures required by mandatory testing program.

The requirements to be met in the technique and management
of the tests that are performed, whether or not the tests themselves *are* made mandatory, is quite a different matter. An HI
test, falsely reported as positive, obviously may lead to the incorrect conclusion that prenatal defects from rubella infection need
not be feared for the child *in utero.* An HI test falsely reported
as negative, on the other hand, may result in unnecessary inter-
ruption of a pregnancy. Now the experiences we have had in
Massachusetts over the years on the results reported on "unknown" bacteriologic and serologic test specimens sent to participating laboratories in our evaluation and approval program,
often for procedures simpler than the HI test for rubella antibodies, show that while many laboratories do excellent work,
some of the laboratories are clearly doing inadequate and unreliable work, at times with disastrous consequences. We can,
therefore, expect from time to time serious errors in the results
of a number of the laboratories, particularly the less experienced,
that even now are being moved to offer the rubella testing service, unless effective evaluation and proficiency testing programs,
administered most logically through the state health department
laboratories, are made available and are used.

There is obvious need for quality control in the performance
of the HI test for rubella antibodies. Technical hazards exist in
the preparation and quantitation of the hemagglutination antigen used, in the age and other qualities of the baby chick red

blood cells used, in the preparation of the serums to be tested, including the all-important removal of nonspecific inhibitors, in the positive and negative controls, and in the temperature maintained for the reagents and during the test itself—to mention some of the hazards. Moreover not only the laboratory director but also the virologists and technicians performing the tests must understand adequately the principles involved, including the interpretation of the results. Only a reasonably sophisticated understanding will endow the laboratory worker with the important built-in sensitivity that warns him what reports on tests that might be released could nevertheless be misleading without an interpretive appraisal. In short, for all these reasons, I can hardly think of a valid argument against the wide use of evaluation and approval programs, which include periodic sets of "unknowns" as a "must," and which are augmented with work shops and other laboratory teaching devices as they are indicated.

Should the evaluations of laboratories performing the rubella tests be mandatory by law? We should be aware, of course, that current regulations at the federal level, which are administered through state agencies, already require proficiency evaluations at least for the independent laboratories involved in work for the medicare program and will soon for work also under the medicaid program. As a result for the independent laboratories, there may or may not be a need for further mandatory legislation. However, the individual state may well elect to supplement the federal proficiency requirements for serologic testing. Certainly each state needs to expand and intensify its own laboratory improvement program. These needs and decisions each state should carefully consider, especially the mandatory inclusion of private and hospital laboratories not covered presently by the federal regulations.

For the hospital as well as for the independent laboratories, we have had for many years in Massachusetts an active and aggressive but voluntary laboratory approval program. This program, when laboratory evaluations reveal difficulties, has always emphasized and rendered when feasible consultative technical help toward improvement rather than censure or punitive action. This has been quite successful, with practically all of the hospital and independent laboratories in the state participating and with the experience of many years confirming the need. It should be expanded to include virology, specifically rubella serologic testing. We would recommend an early trial of such an approach with later conversion to a mandatory program as seems indicated for the individual state. Any such legislative program should be tailored to the particular meeting of the minds that can be achieved through the professional and the lawmaking bodies involved. It must be well-drawn legislation that can realistically be expected to correct the serious shortcomings of individual laboratories.

Chapter 16

CONFERENCE SUMMARY

JAMES E. PRIER

THERE has been, I believe, a peculiar spirit pervading this conference which is not particularly common among meetings of scientists. Perhaps it is born of several things—a sense of urgency; a passion for accuracy in technical matters; a cooperative mobilization of people of many places and varying talents in the steady and persistent pursuit of a common goal. And the result is the distinct impression that a rare event in scientific meetings has occurred—a lack of attempted "one upmanship" by participants, that sort of egomania which seems to be a driving force in the pseudo-competition of science. But, rather, there has been a marked consensus of concern for the only legitimate objective of medicine and biology which is the benefit of humanity.

The history of rubella has been short and dramatic, with the first definition of the real significance of the disease only 28 years old and the identification of the etiologic agent but 7 years past. Considering that the real impetus for concentrated study of rubella was the disastrous results of the 1964 epidemic with possibly 30,000 victims, it seems almost fantasy that we talk today of the practical immunization of the entire susceptible population. But even with such progress there is a note of sadness, for one is led to wonder how it might have been had the knowledge of today been a reality a decade ago—of the human wastage that might have been avoided, and the parental tears that would have had no cause. For it is the nature of our business that we must always hold a reservation in the face of success that perhaps we moved a little too slowly and reached this point in time and achievement just a bit too late.

It is clear that, although there is still much to accomplish to reach the goal of total control of rubella, there is a significant advantage over the situation that existed ten years ago. Today the

141

methods to achieve such an end are available, and the problem is less one of discovery than it is of application. And this can only place us in a more uncomfortable position, for there is no reasonable excuse. The methods are available, if properly applied, to determine the current immune status of each and every individual in the critical category—to identify the 20 percent of the female population of risk. And then to render the necessary prophylaxis that will avoid a subsequent infection.

Serologic testing, however, requires more than just the simple mechanics of a laboratory procedure. If interpretation is to be accurate, the specimens must be taken at the appropriate times, adequate clinical histories must be available, and both laboratorian and clinician must recognize the natural history of the immune response in relation to the specific antibodies being measured. Presence or absence of antibody may not be satisfactory for interpretation, so that quantitative antibody studies may be necessary. Further, the presence or absence of clinical signs of rubella offers no reliable criteria for determining the degree of danger in the case of the pregnant female. It would seem that serologic monitoring of the pregnant female has become unequivocably mandatory.

The isolation of rubella virus from the acute case of rubella can be accomplished, but is not in the category of a routine clinical laboratory procedure. Such a procedure probably has greater diagnostic application for cases of congenital infection. There are several methods available, when adequately controlled, which will permit the monitoring of the long-term virus disseminating congenitally infected child. Combination of isolation technics and appropriate serologic methods can provide an accurate system for identifying the congenitally infected individual, even many months after birth.

The information now available indicates that reliable technical procedures can be applied to justify appropriate handling of the individual clinical case. In the case of early pregnancy with rubella exposure, serologic technics, properly applied, will determine the course to be taken. It must be kept in mind that establishing the negative rubella patient is of equal importance to defining the one that will require subsequent medical attention. There seems little reason to argue that a properly controlled serologic procedure that indicates a definite rise in antibody titer is sufficient cause to consider the termination of pregnancy. But it must be emphasized that such actions have legal as well as medical implications, and, therefore, the accuracy of laboratory procedures is a most critical consideration. Also, it is possible that a single type of serologic test may not be sufficient, so that HI reactions may require CF, or in some cases, even a determination of the globulin characteristic.

A normal epidemiologic pattern dictates that a high incidence period of naturally occurring rubella should present itself in the near future. But such a phenomenon depends upon a more than usual number of susceptibles for virus maintenance and rapid passage, presumably young age groups who have not had previous experience with rubella. It seems logical to presume that the virus can be thwarted in its attempted rampage by interposing an immune young generation of human host. And it appears that the mechanism to create this barrier to the natural history of rubella virus is at hand, if it can be applied with sufficient magnitude.

Programs for checking the immune status of susceptible individuals are feasible, by application of routine serologic screening tests at premarital and prenatal points. The inhibitions to establishing such programs are more fiscal and political than scientific. The public health officer can understand the barriers to the rapid establishment of such programs—but the importance of the objective leads him to question the justification of Federal, state, and local bureaucratic inadequacies.

Services at the community level for detection of rubella antibodies are practical considerations and are to be advocated if suitable control measures are to be effected. A sufficient number of tests must be done to assure competence, and the more complex procedures of CF, fluorescent antibody, IgM, and neutralization should be relegated to reference facilities. Proficiency testing of routine clinical laboratories should and must be made available through state agencies, with appropriate reference and control facilities through cooperation of the federal agency.

Production of adequate supplies of rubella vaccine is progressing at a rapid rate, with an estimation of 6 million doses per month in the near future. This would seem to indicate that material production may become less important than the problem of logistics in supplying vaccine to the recipients. It is probable that the best and most adequate vaccine is yet to be developed, but the consensus at present is that some current products are sufficiently safe and reliable for routine application. Occasional side effects in adults of transient lymphadenopathy and arthralgia may not be highly significant considerations, although it certainly is most desirable to have preparations which do not produce such untoward sequelae. Of most significance is that the antibody response to accepted preparations will provide immunity.

At that point, therefore, there are mechanisms to be put into effect for the diagnosis and prophylaxis of rubella. The individual patient and the general population are both targets for application of diagnostic and immunization procedures. This is not to imply that developmental problems do not remain. Even today, new improvements in HI testing and other serologic procedures are being reported, and others will undoubtedly be forthcoming. Networks of testing facilities must be established. In addition to current information, more data are needed in regard to the phenomenon of congenital chronic rubella infection. Educational programs must be expanded. Legal adjustments in some jurisdictions are indicated to permit appropriate medical handling of known infected pregnant females.

There are other questions yet to be answered. Is it a reliable assumption that attenuated virus has a negligible potential for transmission? Can adequate vaccines be developed that completely eliminate the concern for exposure of the pregnant female? Will studies in time indicate that current concepts of safety in live virus vaccines are naive assumptions?

But when all the titers are determined, and the research logs are closed, and all the vaccine is placed in little vials with neat labels, the most important thing is this: that it will no longer be necessary to deliver to the arms of a young mother a child who is abnormal in mind and body and who may never live to be a man. And that cry of anguish from the deepening shadows of the night will be heard no more.

SUMMARY REPORT OF AD HOC COMMITTEE FOR STANDARDIZATION OF TECHNIQUES

Minimum Information Recommended for Acceptance of Specimens for Laboratory Testing

1. Patient's name and address.
2. Birthdate (age).
3. Sex.
4. Date of onset or exposure to rubella-like illness. Type of exposure (household contact vs. casual contact).
5. Brief clinical summary.
     Rash (onset, distribution, duration)
     Stage of pregnancy (LMP)
     Gamma globulin (amount, date given)
6. Type of specimens.
7. Dates of specimen collection (name and date of collection on each specimen).
8. Name and address of referring physician or laboratory.

Serologic Testing

Bloods collected aseptically by venipuncture. Sera separated using sterile technique and stored in the frozen state.

Outline of Procedures for Collection and Processing of Rubella Diagnostic Specimens

Virus Isolation Attempts

Pharyngeal swabs specimens: Collected with sterile swabs, which are then immersed in approximately 5 ml of Hanks' balanced salt solution (HBSS) containing 1% bovine plasma albumin (BPA) and antibiotics.

Blood specimens collected by venipuncture and heparinized.

Tissue specimens washed with HBSS, weighed, ground and prepared as 10% suspensions in HBSS containing 1% BPA and antibiotics.

145

Specimens inoculated into appropriate cell cultures either as freshly prepared or after storage at −60°C.

References

Virus Isolation: Parkman, P. D., Hopps, H. E., and Meyer, H. M., Jr. Rubella virus, isolation characterization and laboratory diagnosis. *Amer. J. Dis. Child.*, 118:68 (July), 1969.

HI Test Method

Kaolin treatment: Stewart, G. L., *et al.* Rubella-virus hemagglutination inhibition test. *NEJM*, 276:554 (March 9), 1967.

Heparin-MnCl₂ treatment. Cooper, *et al. JAMA*, 207:89-93 (Jan. 6), 1969.

Dextran-SO₄-CaCl₂ treatment. Liebhaber, H. In press.

Complement fixation test methods: Sever, J. L., *et al.* Rubella complement fixation test. *Science*, 148:385 (April 16), 1965; Halonen, J. M.; Ryan, J. M.; and Stewart, J. A. Rubella hemagglutinin prepared with alkaline extraction of virus grown in suspension culture of BHK-21 cells. *Proc. Soc. Exp. Biol. Med.*, 125:162-167 (May), 1967.

Pitfalls of Rubella HI Testing

  I. Operational.
      A. Serum Storage and Handling.
          1. Handle aseptically.
          2. Store frozen (−20°C).
          3. Do *not* discard sera (one year).
      B. Labeling.
          1. Name and number.
          2. *Date.*
      C. Record keeping.
          1. Referring physician's name.
          2. Patient's name.
          3. History of exposure, if any, with date(s) and nature.
 II. Technical.
      A. Do *not* heat serum if inhibitors are to be removed by Heparin MnCl₂ or Dextran-SO₄-CaCl₂ methods.

B. Keep all reagents sterile.

C. Date and identify all reagents by lot number. Each test record should include antigen lot number, cell suspension lot number and diluent lot number.

D. If using a particular HI kit, *do not* substitute reagents or diluents from other kits.

E. ALWAYS run multiple sera from one patient in the same test.

F. Include a positive and negative control in every test and disregard results if controls are off.

G. Run test (i.e. incubation of serum and hemagglutinin) at 4°C.

H. Time of incubation of kaolin with serum should be kept constant.

The committee suggested that primary laboratories, i.e. hospital and clinical pathological laboratories, be proficient in the performance of the HI test only. Primary laboratories should have available a reference laboratory which will usually be a state laboratory or special rubella laboratory and which will be able to perform additional tests as dictated by circumstances.

We would emphasize that primary laboratories should turn to reference laboratories for expert assistance in interpretation of results in difficult situations.

For the diagnosis of various manifestations of rubella, we recommend that the following studies be done.

1. Determination of susceptibility to rubella. Single serum to be tested for HI antibodies.

2. Exposure to possible rubella. Serum to be tested for HI antibodies. Second serum collected at approximately 28 days after exposure to be tested for HI, if first result shows negative or low antibodies.

3. Rash in pregnancy—acute disease. Paired sera collected 7 to 14 days apart to be tested for HI antibodies. Supplement with CH, FA, IgM, and virus isolation when necessary.

4. History of recent rash (retrospective diagnosis). Sera to be sent to reference lab capable of supplementary tests.

5. Congenital rubella syndrome. Sera from infant and mother.

Nasopharyngeal swabs, cerebrospinal fluid and lens for virus isolation. When primary laboratory identifies suspect rubella syndrome by HI test, sera and additional specimens should be sent to reference lab, in order that the diagnosis can be verified and the case can be reported to the National Registry.

6. Possible complications of vaccination. Case and specimens to be referred to reference laboratory.